PARTNERSHIP WORKING IN HEALTH AND SOCIAL CARE

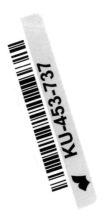

Better partnership working

Series editors: Jon Glasby and Helen Dickinson

About the authors

Jon Glasby is Professor of Health and Social Care and Director of the Health Services Management Centre at the University of Birmingham. A qualified social worker by background, he is Editor-in-Chief of the *Journal of Integrated Care* and an NHS Non-Executive Director at Birmingham Children's Hospital.

Helen Dickinson is Associate Professor of Public Governance at the Melbourne School of Government, University of Melbourne, Australia. Helen has research interests in areas such as governance and collaboration, priority setting and decision making in public services, and the future of the public sector workforce.

PARTNERSHIP WORKING IN HEALTH AND SOCIAL CARE

What is integrated care and
how can we deliver it?

Second edition

First edition published in Great Britain in 2008, reprinted 2009, 2010

This edition published in Great Britain in 2014 by

Policy Press
University of Bristol
6th Floor
Howard House
Queen's Avenue
Clifton
Bristol BS8 1SD
UK
t: +44 (0)117 331 5020
f: +44 (0)117 331 5367
pp-info@bristol.ac.uk
www.policypress.co.uk

North America office:
Policy Press
c/o The University of Chicago Press
1427 East 60th Street
Chicago, IL 60637, USA
t: +1 773 702 7700
f: +1 773 702 9756
sales@press.uchicago.edu
www.press.uchicago.edu

© Policy Press 2014

British Library Cataloguing in Publication Data
A catalogue record for this book is available from the British Library

Library of Congress Cataloging-in-Publication Data
A catalog record for this book has been requested

ISBN 978 1 44731 281 9 paperback

Cover design by Policy Press
Printed and bound in Great Britain by Hobbs, Southampton
Policy Press uses environmentally responsible print partners

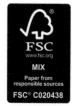

Contents

List of tables, figures and boxes

Tables

Figures

Boxes

List of abbreviations

We have tried to avoid some of the many abbreviations and acronyms used in health and social care. However, a small number of abbreviations are used, including:

CCG	Clinical Commissioning Group
DH	Department of Health
GP	General practitioner
HAZ	Health Action Zone
NHS	National Health Service
PCG/T	Primary Care Group/Trust
PPP	Public–private partnership

All web references in the following text were correct at the time of printing.

Acknowledgements

The authors are grateful to Policy Press and to a number of key colleagues and friends who have allowed us to reproduce their material in this book. Particular thanks go to Chris Skelcher and colleagues for permission to reproduce their Governance Assessment Tool in Box 3.4 and to Annette Hastings for permission to reproduce Tables 4.1 and 4.2. Any personal opinions (and indeed errors) in the book are those of the authors.

Preface

Whenever you talk to people using health and social services, they often assume that the different agencies and professions talk to each other regularly, actively share information and work closely together. Indeed, most people don't distinguish between 'health care' and 'social care' at all, or between individual professions such as 'nursing', 'social work' or 'occupational therapy'. They simply have 'needs' that they want addressing in a professional and responsive manner, ideally by someone they know and trust. How the system is structured behind the scenes could not matter less.

And yet, people working in health and social care know that it *does* matter. No one starts with a blank sheet of paper, and we all have to finds ways of working in a system that was not designed with integration in mind. As this book explains, different parts of health and social care services have evolved over time as largely separate entities, and policy makers, managers and frontline practitioners trying to offer a joined-up service will typically face a series of practical, legal, financial and cultural barriers. This is typically time-consuming and frustrating, and the end result for service users and their families often still does not feel very integrated (no matter how hard the professionals were working to try to produce a joint way forward). As one key commentator suggests, 'you can't integrate a square peg into a round hole' (Leutz, 1999).

When services aren't joined-up, it can result in poor outcomes for everybody – gaps, duplication and wasted time and resources. People using services often express amazement at the number of different people they have to tell their story to. Instinctively, it doesn't feel like a good use of their time or of the skilled professionals who are trying to help them. One part of the system can't often do something until there has been input from another part, and this can lead to all kinds of delays, inefficiencies and missed opportunities.

For staff, it can be surprisingly difficult to find enough time and space to gain a better understanding of how other agencies and professions operate, what they do, what priorities they have and what constraints they face. For someone who went into a caring profession to make a difference, there is nothing more dispiriting than knowing that someone needs a joined-up response but not knowing how to achieve it. In many situations, workers feel they are being asked to help people with complex needs, but with one hand constantly tied behind their back.

For the broader system, this state of affairs seems equally counter-productive. If support is delayed or isn't sufficiently joined-up, it can lead to needs going unmet and to people's health rapidly deteriorating. It then becomes even harder and even more expensive to intervene in a crisis, and this leaves less time and money for other people who are becoming unwell and who need support (creating a vicious cycle). Poor communication, duplication and arguments over who should pay for what all lead to inefficiency, bad feeling and poor outcomes for people using services. In extreme cases, a lack of joint working can also culminate in very serious, tragic situations, such as a child death, a mental health homicide, the abuse of a person with learning difficulties or an older person dying at home alone (see Box 0.1 for but one high profile example). Here, partnership working is quite literally a matter of life and death, and a failure to collaborate can have the most serious consequences for all involved.

Box 0.1: Partnership working as a matter of life or death

Following the tragic death of Peter Connelly (initially known as 'Baby P' in the press), Lord Laming (2009) was asked to produce a national review of progress since his initial investigation into the equally horrific death of Victoria Climbié in the same borough of Haringey (Laming, 2003). As the 2009 review observed (Laming, 2009, para 4.3):

> ... It is evident that the challenges of working across organisational boundaries continue to pose barriers in practice, and that cooperative efforts are often the first to

> suffer when services and individuals are under pressure. Examples of poor practice highlighted in this report include child protection conferences where not all the services involved in a child's life are present or able to give a view; or where one professional disagrees with a decision and their view is not explored in more detail; and repeated examples of professionals not receiving feedback on referrals. As a result of each of these failures, children or young people at risk of neglect or abuse will be exposed to greater danger. The referring professional may also be left with ongoing anxiety and concern about the child or young person. This needs to be addressed if all local services are to be effective in keeping children and young people safe.

For health and social care practitioners, if you are to make a positive and practical difference to service users and patients, most of the issues you face will involve working with other professions and other organisations. For public service managers, partnership working is likely to occupy an increasing amount of your time and your budget, and arguably requires different skills and approaches to those prioritised in traditional single agency training and development courses. For social policy students and policy makers, many of the issues you study and/or try to resolve inevitably involve multiple professions and multiple organisations. Put simply, people do not live their lives according to the categories we create in our welfare services – real-life problems are nearly always messier, more complex, harder to define and more difficult to resolve than this.

Policy context

In response, national and local policy increasingly calls for enhanced and more effective partnership working as a potential solution (see, for example, DH, 2013). While such calls for more joint working can be inconsistent, grudgingly made and/or overly aspirational, the fact remains that collaboration between different professions and different organisations is increasingly seen as the norm (rather than as an exception to the rule). This is exemplified in a recent Welsh policy paper, *Sustainable social services for Wales: A framework for action* (Welsh Assembly Government, 2011, p 11), that argued, 'We want to change the question from "how might we cooperate across boundaries?" to justifying why we are not'. With most new funding and most new policy initiatives, there is usually a requirement that local agencies work together to bid for new resources or to deliver the required service, and various Acts of Parliament place statutory duties of partnership on a range of public bodies. As an example of the growing importance of partnership working, the word 'partnership' was recorded 6,197 times in 1999 in official parliamentary records, compared to just 38 times in 1989 (Jupp, 2000, p 7). When we repeated this exercise for the first edition of this book, we found 17,912 parliamentary references to 'partnership' in 2006 alone (although this fell to 11,319 when removing references to legislation on civil partnerships that was being debated at the time). Since then, there has been a general election, a new government and a series of major spending cuts and pressures, arguably making joint working harder to achieve in practice, but even more important.

In 1998, the Department of Health (DH) issued a consultation document on future relationships between health and social care. Entitled *Partnership in action*, the document proposed various ways of promoting more effective partnerships, basing these on a scathing but extremely accurate critique of single agency ways of working (DH, 1998, p 3):

> All too often when people have complex needs spanning both health and social care good quality services are sacrificed for sterile arguments about boundaries. When this happens people, often the most vulnerable in our society ... and those who care for them find themselves in the no man's land between health and social services. This is not what people want or need. It places the needs of the organisation above the needs of the people they are there to serve. It is poor

> organisation, poor practice, poor use of taxpayers' money – it
> is unacceptable.

Whatever you might think about subsequent policy and practice, the fact that a government document sets out such a strongly worded statement of its beliefs and guiding principles is important. How to move from rhetoric to reality is always the key challenge, but such quotes illustrate that partnership working is no longer an option (if it ever was), but the core business. Under the Coalition government (2010-), this previous language has shifted once again, and most recent policy refers to the importance of 'integrated care' rather than 'partnerships' or 'collaboration'. As the NHS Future Forum (2012, p 3) argues:

> Integration is a vitally important aspect of the experience of health and social care for millions of people. It has perhaps the greatest relevance for the most vulnerable and those with the most complex and long-term needs. We have services to be proud of, and patients in England already receive some of the most joined-up services in the world. However, too many people fall through gaps between services as they traverse journeys of care which are often too difficult for them to navigate themselves. This lack of integration results daily in delays and duplication, wasted opportunities and patient harm. It is time to "mind the gaps" and improve the experience and outcomes of care for people using our services.

While it is not always fully clear what a commitment to more integrated care might mean in practice (see below for further discussion), recent policy seems to be trying to achieve number of different things, including:

- greater *vertical integration* between acute, community and primary care

- greater *horizontal integration* between community health and social care
- more effective joint working between *public health* and local government
- more effective partnerships between the *public, private* and *voluntary sectors*
- more *person-centred care*, with services that feel integrated to the patient.

In response to all this, the time feels right for a second edition of this book. While our overall approach remains the same (see below), key changes include:

- updated references to current policy and practice
- the addition of more recent studies and broader literature
- a greater focus on 'integrated care' under the Coalition government
- new reflective exercises and updated further reading/resources
- updated 'hot topics' (including joint working in a cold climate, the advent of clinical commissioning and the focus on health and well-being).

Aim and ethos of the 'Better partnership working' series

Against this background, this book (and the overall series of which it is part) provides an introduction to partnership working via a series of accessible 'how to' resources (see Box 0.2). Designed to be short and easy to use, they are nevertheless evidence-based and theoretically robust. A key aim is to provide *rigour and relevance* via books that:

- offer practical support to those working with other agencies and professions and provide some helpful frameworks with which to make sense of the complexity that partnership working entails;
- summarise current policy and research in a detailed but accessible manner;

- provide practical but also evidence-based recommendations for policy and practice.

> **Box 0.2: The series at a glance**
>
> - *Partnership working in health and social care* (Jon Glasby and Helen Dickinson)
> - *Managing and leading in inter-agency settings* (Edward Peck and Helen Dickinson)
> - *Interprofessional education and training* (John Carpenter and Helen Dickinson)
> - *Working in teams* (Kim Jelphs and Helen Dickinson)
> - *Evaluating outcomes in health and social care* (Helen Dickinson)

While each book is cross-referenced with others in the series, each is a standalone text with all you need to know as a student, a practitioner, a manager or a policy maker to make sense of the difficulties inherent in partnership working. In particular, the series aims to provide some practical examples to illustrate the more theoretical knowledge of social policy students, and some theoretical material to help make sense of the practical experiences and frustrations of frontline workers and managers.

Although there is a substantial and growing literature on partnership working (see, for example, Hudson, 2000; Payne, 2000; Rummery and Glendinning, 2000; Balloch and Taylor, 2001; 6 et al, 2002; Glendinning et al, 2002a; Sullivan and Skelcher, 2002; Barrett et al, 2005), most current books are either broad edited collections, very theoretical books that are inaccessible for students and practitioners, or texts focusing on partnership working for specific user groups. Where more practical, accessible and general texts exist, these typically lack any real depth or evidence base – in many ways little more than partnership 'cookbooks' that give apparently simple instructions that are meant to lead to the perfect and desired outcome. In practice, anyone who has studied or worked in health and social care knows that partnership working can be both frustrating and messy – even if you follow the so-called 'rules', the end result is often hard to predict, ambiguous and likely to provoke different reactions from different agencies and professions. In contrast, this book series seeks to offer a more 'warts and all' approach to the topic, acknowledging the realities that practitioners, managers and policy makers face in the real world.

Wherever possible the series focuses on key concepts, themes and frameworks rather than on the specifics of current policy and organisational structures (which inevitably change frequently). As a result the series will hopefully be of use to readers in all four countries of the UK. That said, where structures and key policies have to be mentioned, they will typically be those in place in England. While the focus of the series is on public sector health and social care, it is important to note from the outset that current policy and practice also emphasises a range of additional partnerships and relationships, including:

- broader partnerships (for example, with services such as transport and leisure in adult services and with education and youth justice in children's services);
- collaboration not just between services, but between professionals and people who use services;
- relationships between the public, private and voluntary sectors.

As a result, many of the frameworks and concepts in each book may focus initially on public sector health and social care, but will also be relevant to a broader range of practitioners, students, services and service users.

Ultimately, the current emphasis on partnership working and on integration means that everything about public services – their organisation and culture, professional education and training, inspection and quality assurance – will have to change. Against this background, we hope that this series of books is a contribution, however small, to these changes.

Jon Glasby and Helen Dickinson
Health Services Management Centre, University of Birmingham
June 2013

1

What is partnership working and why does it matter?

In almost every walk of life, there is a balance to be struck between the expertise of the single practitioner and the need for cooperation, collaboration and coordination. This is evident in many of life's most stressful events – when you move house, for example, you want both the solicitor and the surveyor to be experts in their respective fields, but you also want all those involved to communicate and to cooperate so that the overall process goes smoothly. Equally, when you fit a new kitchen, you want a qualified gas fitter to install the boiler and an experienced electrician to handle the electrics – if the wrong person tries to do these things then the consequences could be fatal. However, you also want someone in overall control of the project so that there are no unnecessary delays and so that the person tiling the floor comes after the person who has to dig up the floor to lay some pipes. With both these examples – moving house and fitting a kitchen – there is scope for some of the key players to blur the boundary of their role and to sometimes take on broader tasks, but there are also elements of the process that are only appropriate for a qualified expert.

If all this is true of everyday life, it is even more the case in health and social care, where the consequences of getting it wrong can be equally as fatal as the potential for faulty wiring or gas leaks in the examples above. When you move house or fit a kitchen, it can be incredibly frustrating when things go wrong – you can often feel completely powerless to do anything constructive and simply have to wait until problems resolve themselves. If delays leave you without temporary accommodation or without water and power for some time, you incur extra costs, significant disruption to your daily routine and a substantial impact on your quality of life. While the same is true in health and social care, the key difference is the potentially life and death nature of people's contact with formal services. When you are seriously ill and need surgical intervention, waiting or negotiating with busy professionals is often not an option – if you need treatment now, then you really need it. Even in the community, people frequently approach services only reluctantly when they have exhausted every other avenue, and are often tired, scared and in desperate need of someone to help them understand what is happening to them, to think through possible solutions and to support them to get what they need. When you are ill, in pain or facing potentially life-changing events, then being passed from pillar to post by the very services that are meant to be supporting you can be a soul-destroying experience.

Against this background, this chapter explores the growing literature on partnership working and on integrated care in order to produce a practical (albeit tentative) definition of key terms and to help readers think through the different types of relationship they may need with different types of profession and organisation in order to deliver particular outcomes for service users and patients. In the process, this discussion links to some of the frameworks set out later in the book, and includes some practical case studies of health and social care communities that have developed close working relationships, including both positive and negative examples. The chapter concludes by summarising the current policy context, highlighting the problematic nature of the health and social care divide and ways in which this boundary has shifted over time. In the process, this chapter draws out some of the negative implications of the divide for users, practitioners and organisations.

Key terms

Part of the problem with 'partnership working' and 'integration' is that such terms can mean all things to all people. As Leathard (1994, p 5) has vividly observed, this area is a 'terminological quagmire' (demonstrated by the 52 separate terms that Leathard then lists to illustrate her point), a classic example of the 'definitional chaos' described by Ling (2000, p 83). In many ways this is because the issues at stake are complex (and often mean that we have to depart from traditional ways of doing things). However, this confusion is also made worse by the rhetoric in national policy documents (which tend to talk about collaboration in various unspecified ways as being a 'good thing' that leads to all kinds of different and better outcomes for people who use services). While the issue of outcomes is discussed in more detail below and in the final book in the current series, *Evaluating outcomes in health and social care* by Helen Dickinson, there is little doubt that 'collaboration' and 'partnership' became key buzzwords under New Labour, and that 'integrated care' is doing the same under the Coalition government. Other examples from the 1990s include concepts such as 'community', 'empowerment' and 'involvement'. The classic example here is the notion of public–private partnerships (PPPs), which are not necessarily partnerships at all (see below), but which sound much more palatable and much less alien to the public sector because of the use of the word 'partnership' in the title.

In many ways, however, the examples of *community*, *empowerment* and *involvement* above offer some useful insights. While these terms are over-used, used imprecisely and often misused, they all refer to some sort of underlying concept that seems important and worth striving for. We may not know exactly what the term 'empowerment' means, but it feels crucial and we often know it when we see it. In fact, the ambiguity of such terms is arguably a strength as it allows them to mean all things to all people. Similarly, the terms 'partnership working' or 'integrated care' refer to something highly significant and something worth trying to define and understand. Thus, even those commentators who have criticised the lack of precision in current policy still end up having to use some kind of similar term. A good example here is The King's Fund's discussion paper, *Partnerships under pressure*, which quite rightly identifies a number of problems with the term 'partnership' (Banks, 2002, p 5):

> The term "partnerships" is increasingly losing credibility, as it has become a catch-all for a wide range of concepts and a

panacea for a multitude of ills. Partnerships can cover a wide spectrum of relationships and can operate at different levels, from informally taking account of other players, to having a constructive dialogue, working together on a project or service, joint commissioning and strategic alliances.

Despite this, the remainder of the paper provides further definitional clarity, but continues to use the term 'partnership' throughout the rest of the document. In short, terms such as 'partnership working' or 'integration' may not always be very helpful, but they are often the best terms we have, and if they did not exist we would probably have to invent them.

Part of the difficulty in being more precise about key terms is that most writers criticise current approaches, then produce their own definition. While this is understandable, it means that there are a large number of definitions available, and that few commentators mean exactly the same thing by the same terms. For students and for frontline workers this seems unhelpful at best, and runs the risk of complicating further an already complex issue. Rather than repeat the same mistake, this book sets out some examples of basic definitions that we have found helpful (see Box 1.1), and tries to summarise some of the key features that we (and most writers) have in mind when talking about these issues. More important than the actual definition employed, however, is the way in which we distinguish 'partnerships' from other ways of organising public services (discussed in more detail below). For people using this book to study or in practice, the key issue is to check out that, whatever definition is being used, all key partners mean and understand the same thing (and this is a central feature of the subsequent discussion).

Box 1.1: Helpful definitions

In a key introductory textbook, Sullivan and Skelcher (2002) suggest that key features of partnerships are that they:

- involve negotiation between people from different agencies committed to working together over more than the short term;
- aim to secure the delivery of benefits or added value that could not have been provided by any single agency acting alone or through the employment of others (that is, shared goals);
- include a formal articulation of a purpose and a plan to bind partners together.

For Glendinning et al (2002a, p 3), a minimal definition of partnership working requires the involvement of 'at least two agents or agencies with at least some sort of common interests or interdependencies; and would probably also require a relationship between them that involves a degree of trust, equality or reciprocity.'

For the NHS Future Forum (2012), the focus should be on 'integration' or 'integrated care', the true test of which is whether services feel integrated around the patient: 'integration is not about structures, organisations or pathways – it is about better outcomes for patients. The entire health and social care system should embrace a definition of integration that truly puts people at the centre' (p 6).

However, some commentators offer less positive definitions:

- For Alex Scott-Samuel, partnership working is often better described as 'putting mutual loathing aside in order to get your hands on the money' (quoted in Powell and Dowling, 2006, p 308).
- For Powell and Dowling (2006, p 305), partnership working involves 'the indefinable in pursuit of the unachievable'.
- For Thomson and Perry (1998, p 409), 'collaboration is like cottage cheese. It occasionally smells bad and separates easily'.

While we use phrases such as *partnership working*, *joint working*, *collaboration* and *integrated care* interchangeably, these various definitions highlight a number of key issues and principles that are worth stressing (and that readers should bear in mind as they read the rest of this book):

- Behind most definitions is a sense of *added value*, an ability to achieve something together that could not be achieved separately (perhaps encapsulated in the notion of 'the whole being greater than the sum of its parts').
- Also significant is a sense of *reciprocity* (that is, for the relationship to be mutually beneficial, and for some sort of sharing of potential risks or drawbacks).
- Several definitions emphasise some sort of *formal and ongoing relationship* – for some in Box 1.1, collaboration and partnership are clearly a journey and, while they may not yet know where this will lead, the agencies involved must recognise that this is a route they need to travel together.
- In many ways, an acid test is the subsequent experience of *people who use services* – perhaps something is only an effective partnership if it feels like it to people on the receiving end.
- Implicit in several definitions is the notion of partnership and collaboration as *voluntary* in nature – based on trust, equality and recognition of interdependence rather than on compulsion. While we return to the issue of so-called 'forced partnerships' later in the book, a central component of collaboration for us is that individual partners *retain the right of exit* (that is, if the collaboration is not perceived to be delivering desired outcomes for both partners, then they have the right to leave that collaboration). This is clearly very different to other ways of working – in a market-based relationship, for example, there will be a formal contract binding agencies together and often preventing exit, except in very tightly defined circumstances.
- While most literature on collaboration is positive, some definitions (albeit tongue in cheek) hint at *possible negatives* and *cynical motivations*

–

that should warn us against always seeing partnership as a 'good thing' (see below).

Markets, hierarchies and networks: a brief overview

Although it can be difficult to be clear exactly what different commentators mean by terms such as 'partnership' and 'integration', it can help to try to distinguish between these concepts and other ways of delivering public services. Typically, organisational theory distinguishes between services that are organised on the basis of *hierarchies*, *markets* and *networks* (see Box 1.2), and part of the problem is that the term 'partnership' can be used to describe all three. In the UK, many current welfare services began life in the voluntary and community sector, with various 19th-century philanthropists and charities gradually developing new ways of responding to the social problems created by rapid industrialisation and urbanisation. While the development of state welfare is described in more detail elsewhere (see, for example, Hill, 2000; Fraser, 2003), it was often the voluntary sector that pioneered developments such as old-age pensions, child health services, adult education, affordable housing and practical support for older and disabled people, many of which became part of a state-led and publicly funded welfare system following the reforms of the 1940s. In many ways, this was an era of *hierarchy*, with large government departments responsible for a series of (often quite separate) welfare services, each with their own regional and local delivery structures. Authority in such a system was very top-down, with staff at ground level reporting up to a lead officer, who would then report upwards.

From the late 1970s, a series of national and international economic crises prompted a radical rethink, and the Conservative governments of Margaret Thatcher (1979-90) began a process of *market-based reform*. According to this ideology, a very large public sector had become massively inefficient, consuming too much of the nation's resources and serving the interests of staff and welfare professionals rather than people receiving services. In response, public services were reformed

–

7

according to market principles, with the public sector increasingly focused on purchasing services from a growing range of public, private and voluntary organisations, rather than providing them all itself 'in-house'. Thus, in the National Health Service (NHS), a 'purchaser–provider split' meant that health authorities were increasingly to pay for the hospital services provided to local people by a series of new and more self-financing hospital trusts. In social care, the community care reforms of the early 1990s increasingly saw social workers as assessors and care managers, identifying and meeting needs from a menu of services (that could be provided by a range of different organisations and not just by in-house social care services). In a market-based system like this, the emphasis was very much on assessing needs (both of the population and of the individual) and securing the services to meet those needs from the best available supplier. While 'best' here could include considerations of cost, quality and responsiveness to service user needs, there was arguably a tendency to focus on cost as the main criterion. Under a market, moreover, service providers have a strong incentive to change their behaviour in order to be efficient and competitive, but there is also a risk of increased costs and complexity when trying to establish and manage the market, to judge quality and to ensure standards. Where services are very specialist, there can often be a risk of a single provider monopolising all provision (which then prevents competition and can remove incentives to remain cost-effective and efficient). More generally, those services better able to adapt to the market also tend to out-survive competitors who struggle to change. While this can remove some poor quality services, it can also lead to a situation where larger and larger companies take over the majority of suppliers and where small organisations can no longer afford to keep up.

Under New Labour, interest grew in the concepts of partnerships and *networks*. In many ways, this was a response to the practical implications of the changes of the 1980s and the 1990s. As a result of previous market reforms, public services became increasingly fragmented, with a growing split between commissioners of services and providers from the public, private and voluntary sectors. This is described by Sullivan and Skelcher (2002, pp 15-20) in terms of 'the hollowed-out state', with the government continuing to be responsible for identifying what services were needed and much less involved in delivering this itself. At the very time when policy was starting to focus on more complex, cross-cutting social problems, therefore, mechanisms for responding to such need were increasingly diverse and fragmented. Against this background, the solution, perhaps unsurprisingly, was the notion of 'joined-up solutions to joined-up problems', with a much greater emphasis on interagency working and partnership as a means of coordinating something of a patchwork quilt of services. Within this context, the term *network* is often used to describe a way of organising based much more on informal relationships, trust and reciprocity (see Box 1.2), although in practice it is broadly agreed that hierarchies were not replaced by networks.

More recently, policy under the Coalition government has been difficult to categorise. When the initial 2010 White Paper, *Equity and excellence*, was published (DH, 2010), it was seen by many as likely to lead to a greater role for markets and for competition. This was actively resisted by a range of patient and professional groups, leading to widespread political, media and public debate (for a key overview, see Timmins, 2012). As opposition increased, a series of changes were introduced to stress the importance of delivering 'integrated care' (and that this should be understood as meaning services and support that are integrated around the patient, irrespective of how these services are organised behind the scenes). According to one interpretation, this could be a key statement of policy intent, transcending previous debates about hierarchies, markets and networks. On the other hand, it could simply be a pragmatic way of trying to promote a degree of market-based reform without causing too much fragmentation or incurring too much political hostility. At the time of writing, it feels too early to tell, although the policy rhetoric itself could prove helpful to local practitioners and services seeking a degree of official 'permission' to develop new, more integrated approaches.

Box 1.2: Hierarchies, markets and networks

A *hierarchy* is often a single organisation (perhaps a large bureaucracy), with top-down rules, procedures and statutes that govern how the organisation works.

In contrast, a *market* involves multiple organisations exchanging goods and services based on competition and price.

A *network* is often seen as lying in between these two approaches, with multiple organisations coming together more informally, often based on interpersonal relationships or a shared outlook (Thompson et al, 1991; 6 et al, 2006).

As a helpful shorthand, Rodríguez et al (2007, p 158) have caricatured these approaches as being about:

- rules (hierarchy)
- incentives (market)
- interactions (network).

Markets, hierarchies and networks: the more complex reality

Of course, the problem with the brief overview above is that it runs the risk of over-simplifying a more complex reality. Often organisations do not solely interact according to one of these modes, and it is possible to get hierarchies within markets and market-like networks. While the distinction between 1940s-1970s hierarchy, 1980s markets and post-1997 networks is a useful shorthand, it portrays the evolution of services in a very linear way. In practice, we believe that the shift from hierarchies to markets to networks may be more cyclical. Thus, over time traditional hierarchies run the risk of being seen as bureaucratic, very large/expensive and unresponsive to need. While there is no inherent reason why a hierarchy should be like this, the temptation in our political system has been to break up these hierarchies and to turn them into markets, thus using choice, competition and 'customer power' to make services change. Over time, markets can be seen as creating too much fragmentation, and networks become a more attractive concept – bringing together different stakeholders to work in new, more cross-cutting ways. However, as the issue at stake rises up the political agenda, it can reach a stage where it is deemed to be so important that we no longer trust networks to handle it, and we quickly turn it back into a hierarchy (which we feel we can manage and control more directly). From here the cycle begins again.

While this sounds abstract, some more concrete examples in Box 1.3 show how this can happen in practice. Moreover, this is an important debate because of our tendency to use words such as 'partnership' very imprecisely to refer to hierarchies, markets and networks all at the same time (see Box 1.4). Thus, many current health and social care 'partnerships' are actually hierarchies – they may bring together health and social care, but they do so in large, public sector bureaucracies with a chief executive and a board, a senior management team and all the systems and processes of a standard hierarchical organisation. Equally, some market-based relationships – for example, PPPs – are (wrongly) described as 'partnerships', perhaps because they can involve long-term relationships but also because it sounds more attractive and politically acceptable. Similarly, many networks share many features with the key definitions in Box 1.1 above, and represent a particular form of partnership.

Box 1.3: Cyclical changes in the way we organise services

Arguably, health, and to a lesser extent, social care, have a cultural preference for hierarchy, yet there has been a growing distrust of bureaucracy and over-centralisation. Over time, a number of initiatives have arisen as networks, yet have quickly become so important that we have turned them back into hierarchies. At the same time, some hierarchies have seemed so large and potentially inefficient that we have broken them up via market mechanisms. Examples include:

- *Changes in mental health services*, where initial community mental health teams (which were very loose, informal and bottom-up

---

collaborations) have become increasingly hierarchical as mental health has become more of a political priority. Under recent policy, there is detailed guidance as to what kind of teams we need, staff numbers and caseloads, in a much more hierarchical, managed system.

- In *child protection*, a similar shift from network-based area child protection arrangements to much more hierarchical safeguarding children boards took place following a number of high profile child deaths and a landmark inquiry by Lord Laming (2003) into the death of Victoria Climbié.

- *Health Action Zones* (HAZs) often began as networks to bring people together to develop innovative responses to cross-cutting problems such as health inequalities. Over time, these initiatives were given more and more central targets, were subjected to tighter central control and began to appoint their own 'directors'. As they began to be perceived as 'not delivering' or as too large and inefficient, many HAZs began to contract out their work to the market.

Box 1.4: 'Partnership working': meaning all things to all people

Some health and social care partnerships are actually hierarchies – a Care Trust or a mental health partnership trust, for example. While we discuss the example of the integrated mental health trust created in Somerset in Chapter 2, this was initially seen as a ground-breaking example of collaboration and partnership. With hindsight, it was actually a network in the process of turning into a hierarchy (albeit an integrated one), and the language used to describe this important innovation should perhaps have been more precise.

The PPP Forum is 'a private sector industry body for public private partnerships delivering UK infrastructure. Its aims are to: demonstrate the success the private sector is achieving in delivering modern public services infrastructure; engage with government departments and related organisations to develop infrastructure procurement policy and contracts; take part in public debate and present an informed and business based perspective on infrastructure procurement and the surrounding issues' (see www.pppforum.com).

In the NHS, several medical specialities have developed clinical networks, with professionals in areas such as cancer, heart disease and diabetes coming together as a network to develop more patient-focused care across primary and secondary healthcare services (for a recent Scottish example, see www.nsd.scot.nhs.uk/services/nmcn/index.html). However, some approaches talk of 'managed clinical networks', and it isn't always clear what blend of hierarchy and network this implies.

Overall, the upshot of all this is twofold:

• When people talk about partnership and integration, they often mean very different things by the same terms. As a result, it is crucial to be abundantly clear about the kind of relationship being talked about.
• Ultimately, what matters most is what you are trying to achieve for service users and for your organisation. Only when you are clear about what you want to achieve can you move on to consider who you need to work with and what kind of relationships you may need. This is discussed in further detail in Chapter 4, with various frameworks to help clarify these issues and to guide decision making.

Why does partnership working matter?

Just as there are a wide range of definitions of 'partnership', so too there are a myriad of checklists that set out the supposed advantages of partnership working (see Box 1.5 for some of many potential examples). Unfortunately, such lists tend to be unremittingly positive, emphasising perceived benefits without citing any evidence for the claims made and without listing any of the potential negatives. The extent to which current evidence is able to identify whether partnerships are effective (and if so, for whom and under which circumstances) is explored later in Chapters 2 and 3 (as well as in another book in this series, *Evaluating outcomes in health and social care*, by Helen Dickinson). While doing some things together seems more sensible than doing them separately, it is actually quite hard to understand whether this is true and, if so, why, how and in what circumstances. Certainly, many of the claims made in Box 1.5 (although they intuitively feel credible) are not based on clear-cut and unambiguous evidence, and approaching a topic such as partnership working with a healthy scepticism may be a good way forward. Even more important than this, however, is the need to place the current emphasis on partnership working/integrated care in a broader context in order to understand where it has come from and why it has developed the way it has.

Often, when the world changes, we like to think it is because of the power of ideas – because somebody somewhere has had a vision of how things could be different and has convinced enough people to make this start to happen. Unfortunately, all the available evidence suggests that the power of ideas can be limited by what it seems possible to think. In other words, people are predisposed to have and accept new ideas by the context in which they live and work – by the unwritten rules about why life, the universe and everything is the way it is. Thus, at any given time, some ideas and changes seem feasible and/or desirable, but this is governed by the current economic, political, social and cultural context in which we are located.

Box 1.5: Why work in partnership?

For the Audit Commission (1998, p 9), there are five main reasons why agencies develop partnerships:

- To deliver co-ordinated packages of services to individuals
- To tackle so-called "wicked issues" [that is, cross-cutting, complex problems where we do not really know the best way of responding to the issue at stake]
- To reduce the impact of organisational fragmentation and minimise the impact of any perverse incentives that arise from it

---

- To bid for, or gain access to, new resources, and
- To meet a statutory requirement.

For Payne (2000, p 41), there are six purposes for multiprofessional work: bringing together skills; sharing information; achieving continuity of care; apportioning and ensuring responsibility and accountability; coordination in planning resources; and coordination in delivering resources for professionals to apply for the benefit of service users.

For the DH (1998, p 5):

> Those most likely to suffer from the failure of the current system are the most vulnerable – frail older people, adults or children with mental health problems, learning or physical disabilities. They require support from both health and social services because of the changing and ongoing nature of their needs. Our proposals ... are designed to help those most in need by ensuring better delivery of the services they want when they want them.

For the NHS Future Forum (2012, p 10), integrated care is needed in order to improve services that too often operate in isolation:

> Sadly, in our listening exercise across England we have been told repeatedly that the system, as it stands, often does not deliver the integrated package of care that people ... need. It doesn't deliver their desired outcomes either. There are often wide gaps between services, particularly between primary and secondary medical care, and between health and social care. The often inefficient and unreliable transitions between services result in duplication, delays, missed opportunities and safety risks. Designing and delivering more joined-up and patient-centred services offers the hope of improving patient experience, safety, quality, outcomes and value.

In terms of partnership working and integration, the dramatic rise in the importance of this topic can seem at first glance like a vindication for the power of ideas. If we revisit the 1998 *Partnership in action* quote from the Preface, one interpretation is of a government that has diagnosed a key problem in current services and that is taking a decisive and principled stand to put things right (DH, 1998, p 3):

> All too often when people have complex needs spanning both health and social care good quality services are sacrificed for sterile arguments about boundaries. When this happens people, often the most vulnerable in our society … and those who care for them find themselves in the no man's land between health and social services. This is not what people want or need. It places the needs of the organisation above the needs of the people they are there to serve. It is poor organisation, poor practice, poor use of taxpayers' money – it is unacceptable.

While this is a powerful rationale, an additional explanation is that the context is currently right for partnership working to be seen as a 'good thing' and as the best way forward for health and social care services. This is a complex issue beyond the scope of the current book series (although for a more detailed account of these changes in an international context, see Glasby and Dickinson, 2009). For present purposes, Box 1.6 sets out some of the key factors that we feel have contributed to the current emphasis on partnership working and integration, although this list is neither definitive nor uncontested.

Box 1.6: Factors promoting a focus on partnership working and integrated care

When a new way of working becomes a core feature of policy (in the UK and in many other developed countries), it is often the result of a series of wider and interrelated political, economic and social factors. For example, the current emphasis on partnership working could be variously attributed to some combination of the following factors:

- the increased fragmentation of services following the implementation of various market-based approaches to public services;
- the emphasis placed on 'customer satisfaction' by current political philosophies;
- the growth of various civil rights movements (around 'race', gender and disability), with service user-led organisations increasingly calling for services that enable them to lead chosen lifestyles (and for services that fit their lives, not the other way round);
- demographic changes (with older, more diverse and more mobile populations) and advances in medicine and technology, leading to a need to deliver services in new and more cost-effective ways;
- rising public expectations and a growing challenge to traditional professional power;
- the need for a political narrative as to how public services can continue to meet growing levels of need in an era of financial restraint and how to strike an appropriate balance between competition and collaboration;
- at a local level, managers seeking to bring about major service change can sometimes find concepts such as 'partnerships' or 'integrated care' useful as they have a positive connotation, are hard to argue against and help create a vision for frontline staff.

Again, this is much more than an academic exercise – such issues matter because they help to explain why partnership working is being promoted, why frontline practitioners experience some of the frustrations they do, why different policies can often seem contradictory in nature and why it is so difficult to evaluate partnership working. Put simply, if people working in partnerships have very different (and often subconscious) motivations for doing so, then we should not be surprised if the results are ambiguous, unclear and contested.

Policy context

In many ways, both current and previous attempts to promote more effective partnerships arise directly out of the underlying assumptions that underpin our current welfare system (for an overview, see Means and Smith, 1998; Means et al, 2003; Glasby and Littlechild, 2004; Glasby, 2012a). Under the 1940s legislation that set up the current welfare state, it was assumed that it was possible to distinguish between people who were *sick* (that is, people we see as having *health needs* that are met by the NHS free at the point of delivery) and people who were merely *frail or disabled* (who we see as having *social care needs* that fall under the remit of local authority adult social services and that are frequently subject to a means test and to user charges). This underlying distinction then results in two separate agencies with very different structures, priorities, financial systems and ways of working, and all the subsequent complexities that partnership working entails (see Box 1.7 for a summary of key differences between health and social care over time). There have been many attempts to overcome this boundary – from joint consultative committees in the 1970s to hospital discharge protocols in the 1990s, and from local agreements over the boundary between home care and district nursing to a raft of national guidance on the difference between long-term care, free personal care and NHS continuing healthcare (for a more detailed discussion, see Glasby and Littlechild, 2004). However, the fact remains that this divide continues to exist and continues to cause problems for policy makers, practitioners and service users alike. While recent policy has become much more sophisticated at hiding and blurring the health and social care divide, its influence is no less profound than it ever was.

Box 1.7: The health and social care divide

- Healthcare is accountable nationally to the Secretary of State for Health; social care is part of local government and accountable to locally elected councillors.
- Healthcare is free at the point of delivery; (adult) social care often entails a means test and user charges.
- Healthcare tends to be based on general practitioner (GP) registration (which is often based on catchment areas around individual practices); social care is based on strict local authority geographical boundaries.
- Healthcare is often dominated by medicine and looks to the sciences for its education and training; social care is much more influenced by the social sciences.
- Healthcare often focuses on curing the individual; social care places greater emphasis on seeing the individual in context and potentially intervening socially and politically rather than always individually.
- Following the 2010 general election, the overall NHS budget has been protected, while adult social care has faced substantial cuts (as part of broader cuts to the overall local government budget).

In children's services, the nature of the debate is slightly different. While the health and social care divide continues to be a source of potential fragmentation, a more prominent fault line is between the education system (with its emphasis on attainment and qualifications) and social care (with its emphasis on protection and well-being). As with adult health and social care, such approaches are arguably two sides of the same coin, and it would seem as if feeling safe and happy should be a fundamental building block for subsequent educational attainment. However, this is not the way our system is structured, and both education and children's social care have historically been governed by different government departments, different organisational structures, different financial systems and different cultures and values. Nowhere is this more apparent than in recent performance measures – with schools assessed on the educational achievements of their pupils, there is an incentive built in to the system to work with those pupils most likely to score well in their examinations. While education may therefore be trying to raise the number of children passing their GCSEs with grades A–C, social care is working to protect and include many children and young people who could be seen as 'dragging results down' in a system geared to performance alone. Although this is a massive over-simplification of a much more complicated reality, it is a recognisable over-simplification and may contain more than a degree of truth behind the parody.

However, we should be careful about seeing the emphasis on partnership working as the sole product of the problematic health/social care or education/children's social care divide. No matter how their services are structured or funded, most, if not all, developed countries are struggling with the same issues (see, for example, Johri et al, 2003; Leichsenring and Alaszewski, 2004; Kodner, 2006; Glasby and Dickinson, 2009), and even the briefest of trawls across the experience of other systems suggests that there is no such thing as the perfect organisational structure (see below). No matter where we put the boundary, organisational divisions will always exist, and it depends on your perspective as to whether current boundaries are more or less helpful. As Leutz (1999) has argued in an often-cited commentary on integration, 'your integration is my fragmentation'. Wherever the boundary is located, the trick is in how best to manage it and limit any negative implications for people who use services (and it is this that lies behind the current book and the wider book series).

Arising out of this policy context, health and social care in the early 21st century are developing and drawing on a range of different forms of collaboration as they seek to meet the demands being made of them. Although Box 1.8 provides some of the more prominent examples, we should again guard against the danger of seeing partnership and integration as inherently 'a good thing'. While each health and social care community is trying to find the best and most locally appropriate way forward through the complexities they face, there are many negative as well as positive examples (see Box 1.9), and the evidence base behind current collaborations is thin to say the least. Against this background, the remainder of this book (and the wider series of which it is part) seeks to summarise the key messages from research and to provide a series of broader theoretical frameworks so that busy students, practitioners, managers and policy makers can make as much sense as possible of these difficult issues and hopefully be better equipped as they work with partner agencies. However, underlying the remainder of the book and the series as a whole is the issue of *outcomes* – being clear about what health and social care partners are trying to achieve for their own organisations and for people who use services, about which options are available to them, and about which partnerships and with whom may work best in any given situation. Ultimately, this can be paraphrased as a key question that remains largely unanswered in the current policy context, and that all potential 'partners' would do well to ask themselves – if partnership/integration is the answer, what is the question?

Box 1.8: Examples of current partnerships

Under the 1999 Health Act, health and social care can use one or more of three 'flexibilities' (the ability to pool funding, create an integrated service provider and/or to nominate one partner as a lead commissioner) (for the results of an early national evaluation, see Glendinning et al, 2002b).

Under the 2001 Health and Social Care Act, health and social care communities can create a Care Trust – a single integrated organisation. These are essentially NHS bodies with social care responsibilities delegated to them, and could either focus on providing services (for example, building on a previous NHS mental health trust) or on providing and commissioning (for example, building on a previous NHS Primary Care Trust [PCT]). Unpopular with local government, there were only ever a small number of Care Trusts – and commissioning-based Care Trusts have been replaced by new Clinical Commissioning Groups (for an introductory textbook, see Glasby and Peck, 2003; for a more recent update, see Miller et al, 2011).

In children's services, a children's trust brings together all services for children and young people, underpinned by a duty to cooperate set out

---

in the 2004 Children Act. In addition, key policies for joining up children's services include a common assessment framework, work to develop the role of a lead professional and greater information sharing (for the results of a national evaluation of children's trusts, see University of East Anglia, 2007). Having previously created a separate director of children's services, many councils are now trying to re-combine their children and adult services (often with an overall 'director of people'-type role).

Short of such structural solutions, other collaborations take the form of joint appointments between health and social care, integrated management structures, single assessment processes and 'one-stop shop' entry points into the health and social care system. As but one example, Wistow and Waddington (2006) review the experience of a London borough with a single PCT chief executive and director of social services, although this experiment was short-lived.

Following the 2008 Darzi review, the DH created a series of integrated care pilots in 16 locations to explore different ways of providing more joined-up care (for an evaluation, see RAND Europe/Ernst & Young, 2012).

Under the 2007 Local Government and Involvement in Health Act, health and social care have a duty to carry out an annual Joint Strategic Needs Assessment (for an early study, see Ellins and Glasby, 2008).

Following the 2012 Health and Social Care Act, responsibility for public health has passed to local government. New Clinical Commissioning Groups (CCGs) are also coming together with the local authority to form new Health and Well-Being Boards and to create new Health and Well-being Strategies for their local area (Humphries et al, 2012).

Box 1.9: The negatives of partnership working

In Wiltshire, high-profile financial difficulties and an apparent breakdown in communication between health and social care led to the dismantling of long-standing partnership arrangements and high-profile media discussion (see, for example, O'Hara, 2006).

In Cornwall, inspectors found evidence of abuse and poor practice in a number of learning disability services. Although these were provided by a 'partnership trust', the inspectors concluded that 'working relations between the trust and Cornwall County Council have been poor for a considerable time' (Healthcare Commission/CSCI, 2006, p 7).

In Manchester, an abuse scandal in a newly formed Care Trust prompted significant criticism from national inspectors, who questioned the readiness of previous organisations to form a Care Trust, expressed concerns over relations between the Care Trust and other partners, and argued that the process of forming a Care Trust may have detracted senior management time away from service issues and quality of care (CHI, 2003).

In Barking and Dagenham, the local authority and PCT had initially appointed a single chief executive of the PCT/executive director of health and social care, yet this broke down after a negative star rating of the PCT amid significant negative media coverage (see, for example, Batty, 2003).

Interestingly, some of these examples of negative aspects of partnership working relate to issues of *process* (how well agencies work together), while others refer to negative *outcomes* for service users. This is a key distinction that recurs throughout this book and that is explored in more detail below.

Reflective exercises

1. As a private individual, think of situations where you have been trying to get a good outcome from a situation that needs a number of individuals/agencies working together. This could be, for example, moving house, organising a wedding, or dealing with insurance companies after a car crash. What kind of outcome did you manage to achieve, and how coordinated was the process? How did it feel to be dependent on other people's systems and approaches, and what helped/hindered? Compared to some of the situations that occur in health and social care, these are actually fairly simple examples, yet even here your experience may sometimes have been difficult, frustrating, dispiriting and less than optimal.

2. Write a definition of the terms 'partnership working' and 'integrated care'. How similar are your definitions to some of the debates summarised in this book? Compare your definition with that of a colleague from a different professional background, exploring any key differences. What implications might this have for how you work together?

3. Think about a local organisation where you work or have read about. What kinds of relationships does it have with different partners? To what extent would you describe the agency or its partners as operating within hierarchies, markets or networks?

4. Think about a service user from your caseload or that you have read about in the trade press. What needs do they have and how many different agencies/professions might be involved? How easily do different parts of their life translate into service definitions such as 'health' or 'social care'? How well do current services respond to the person's needs? What needs to be different in future?

5. In a situation where you have worked with somebody from a different organisational or professional background, how easy was it to work together? What outcomes did you achieve together that you couldn't have delivered by yourself? Was any extra benefit worth the investment of time and resources it may have taken to create

—

a joint response? How does this make you feel about working with others again in future? If possible, compare a situation where you produced a good outcome and a case with a less positive outcome.

Note: All the reflective exercises in this book assume that practitioners will be able to draw on first-hand experiences from their work. For students who may not yet have experienced such issues, these exercises work just as well if you apply them to a case study from the trade press/ newspapers or to any other interagency or collaborative situation – for example, playing in a sports team, organising a student society or coming together to do group work on your course.

Further reading and resources

For official health and social care policy, relevant websites include:

- Department of Health: www.dh.gov.uk
- Department for Education: www.education.gov.uk
- Department for Communities and Local Government: www. communities.gov.uk

For guidance on good practice and on 'what works' in health and social care, see the National Institute for Health and Clinical Excellence (NICE) (www.nice.org.uk) and the Social Care Institute for Excellence (www.scie.org.uk).

In terms of the health and social care professions, relevant professional bodies include:

- Association of Directors of Adult Social Services: www.adss.org.uk
- Association of Directors of Children's Services: www.adcs.org.uk
- British Association/College of Occupational Therapists: www.cot. org.uk
- The Chartered Society of Physiotherapy: www.csp.org.uk
- College of Social Work: www.collegeofsocialwork.org

- National Association of Primary Care: www.napc.co.uk
- NHS Alliance: www.nhsalliance.org
- NHS Confederation: www.nhsconfed.org
- Royal College of General Practitioners: www.rcgp.org.uk
- Royal College of Nursing: www.rcn.org.uk

Key introductory textbooks on health and social care partnerships include:

- Barrett et al's (2005) *Interprofessional working in health and social care*
- Glasby's (2012a) *Understanding health and social care*
- Glendinning et al's (2002a) *Partnerships, New Labour and the governance of welfare*
- Meads et al's (2005) *The case for interprofessional collaboration in health and social care*
- Pollard et al's (2010) *Understanding interprofessional working in health and social care*
- Sullivan and Skelcher's (2002) *Working across boundaries*

Helpful policy papers include:

- Curry and Ham's (2010) *Clinical and service integration: The route to improved outcomes*
- Glasby et al's (2011) *All in this together? Making best use of health and social care resources in an era of austerity*
- Goodwin et al's (2012) *Integrated care for patients and populations: Improving outcomes by working together*

Relevant articles can be found in journals such as:

- The UK's *Journal of Integrated Care* (with a helpful focus on the practice implications of recent research and policy)
- The *International Journal of Integrated Care* (free online journal available via www.ijic.org)

2

What does research tell us?

While partnership and integration are increasingly seen as a 'good thing', the evidence base underpinning such assumptions is remarkably thin. Given ongoing commitments to evidence-based policy and practice, this rather aspirational approach to partnership working and integration seems ironic to say the least – and we still know very little about the extent to which partnerships can deliver outcomes that other approaches cannot. In particular, much of the early partnership literature has tended to focus on how well agencies and professions are working together (or not), exploring the extent to which partners feel that they have a good relationship, trust each other and communicate regularly. While these are important issues, they concentrate very much on issues of *process* (how are we working together?), not on issues of *outcome* (does this make any difference to people using services?). As a result, despite a growing literature, our knowledge about what works for whom and in which circumstances remains extremely patchy (for more detailed discussion, see *Evaluating outcomes in health and social care* by Helen Dickinson, in this series).

Against this background, this chapter reviews the claims made for partnership working, and questions the extent to which they are evidence-based. In the course of this discussion, the chapter summarises the literature on what helps and hinders partnership working, and cites practical examples from various health and social care communities. In the process, the chapter also draws on evidence from private sector mergers and acquisitions, questioning the extent to which structural change alone is able to deliver different outcomes, and raising important questions about recent policy.

Neglect of outcomes

As suggested in Chapter 1, much of the literature is extremely positive about the potential outcomes of partnership working for service users. Despite this, the fact remains that we know very little about the impact of partnership working, and many of the claims made above seem more faith- than evidence-based. As Box 2.1 suggests, most attempts to review the literature on the outcomes of partnership conclude that too few studies focus on issues of impact and effectiveness, and that our evidence base is surprisingly under-developed. For Powell and Dowling (2006, p 305), partnerships are 'the indefinable in pursuit of the unachievable'; while 'there is no shortage of advice on how to "do" partnerships ... with lists of drivers, building blocks, and components...,, the validity and reliability of this input into "evidence-based" policy making is less clear'.

Box 2.1: Neglect of outcomes in the partnership literature

In 2003, a systematic review of the factors promoting/hindering joint working concluded that:

> Disappointingly, the vast majority of the studies in the review focused their attention on the process of joint working and the perceptions of those involved as to its success. Very few of the studies looked at either the prior question of why joint work should be seen as a "good thing" and therefore why it should be done, or at the subsequent question of what difference joint working made. This makes the literature somewhat circular, and almost silent on the question of effectiveness. The circularity of the literature led us to the disappointing conclusion that our knowledge ... has hardly moved on since the studies carried out in the late 1970s and early 1980s. (Cameron and Lart, 2003, p 15)

In 2012, an updated version of this review revealed similar results, adding that:

> The evidence base underpinning joint and integrated working remains less than compelling. It largely consists of small-scale evaluations of local initiatives which are often of poor quality and poorly reported. No evaluation studied for the purpose of this briefing included an analysis of cost-effectiveness. There is an urgent need to develop high-quality, large-scale research studies that can test the underpinning assumptions of joint and integrated working in a more robust manner and assess the process from the perspective of service users and carers as well as from an economic perspective. (Cameron et al, 2012, p 1)

In 2004, a review by Dowling et al (p 315) concluded that:

> The present authors' search of the literature has revealed the rudimentary state of the art of conceptualising, measuring and demonstrating the success of partnerships.... [Of studies included], only a few investigated whether specific partnerships had produced successful outcomes and the results were ambiguous even in these.... Thus ... knowledge of whether partnerships "work" – in the sense of producing benefits to those who pay for, provide or use services – remains very limited.

In 2010, a review of public health partnerships identified similar results:

> This article reports on the findings from a systematic review of the impact of partnership working on public health, and considers whether these partnerships have delivered better health outcomes for local/target populations. It finds that there is little evidence that partnerships have produced better health outcomes for local/target populations or reduced health inequalities. (Perkins et al, 2010, p 101)

Local examples

Often, the literature on integrated care seeks to overcome some of these limitations by drawing lessons from local examples and experiences. This is an important form of evidence, and can provide significant insights not available anywhere else. Such studies also shed light on the importance of local context, with different approaches seeming to work better for different areas according to local history, geography and relationships. For present purposes, this section focuses on three main studies/examples: Somerset, Torbay and the national Integrated Care Organisation pilots. The advantage of this approach is that it allows evidence from local practice and experience to inform the debate. Of course, one of the potential disadvantages is that areas with a strong reputation for joint working aren't always representative of health and social care communities elsewhere, and the lessons learned may not always be transferable.

Somerset (Peck et al, 2002)

Following a 1996 review of mental health services, Somerset Health Authority and Somerset County Council took the then unique step of establishing a joint commissioning board and an integrated health and social care provider. Equally unusually, Somerset took the brave step of commissioning a two-and-a-half-year evaluation of these innovations, choosing to make the lessons learned available nationally and publicly. In many ways, Somerset's vision then set the future trend for national policy and for other services, and the changes were subsequently taken up in mental health services and beyond across the country. However, from the beginning, the results of the Somerset study were ambiguous, and different interpretations exist as to the extent to which the integration was a success, and the insights into partnership working that this example provides (see Box 2.2).

> **Box 2.2: Different interpretations of 'success'**
>
> In 2000, the government's 10-year blueprint for health services, *The NHS Plan* (DH, 2000, p 71), quoted the Somerset Partnership NHS and Social Care Trust as an example of good practice, citing benefits for service users such as the existence of a single care plan, a single key worker and a unified multidisciplinary team.
>
> In the subsequent independent evaluation published two years later, the researchers identified evidence of an initial reduction in job satisfaction, morale and role clarity, little change in levels of user satisfaction, and ambiguous results for service users (with some improvements in coordination but also concerns about the potential closure of buildings and a loss of therapeutic/support groups) (Peck et al, 2002). Although sympathetic to what was being undertaken in Somerset and respectful of the extent to which such major change could take place with relatively little upheaval, the research presented a very different picture to that of the 2000 *NHS Plan* (DH, 2000).

While the changes in Somerset were impressive in their scope and seemed to bring about some positive changes for service users, the findings of the evaluation were nuanced. While service user satisfaction remained relatively high and consistent throughout the study, staff morale declined significantly in the short term, with concerns about workload, about a perceived loss of influence for numerically small professions and about the nature and identity of the new organisation. Although there was some evidence that service users felt that they had fewer problems keeping themselves occupied by the end of the study, it is hard to know if this was the result of the integration per se, and the problem of trying to unpick what might have happened anyway without the creation of the new Trust remains. At the same time, service user concerns about the quality of acute inpatient care, about a lack of alternatives to hospital and about a lack of respect from some staff members remained similar over time (for a summary of key findings, see Box 2.3).

Box 2.3: Sample findings from the Somerset Partnership NHS and Social Care Trust

- In the short term, staff found that job satisfaction, morale and role clarity reduced, although this had levelled off and in some cases reversed by the end of the study.
- While the mental health status of service users improved during this period, it is not clear whether this was attributable to the integration itself.
- While coordination improved, some users were concerned about a loss of therapeutic/support groups due to changes in the use of buildings.
- There were continued concerns about lack of alternatives to hospital in a crisis, the extent to which users were involved in negotiating care plans and the attitudes of some staff.
- While there were some improvements for carers, problems continued to exist with identifying, involving and providing information to carers.

Source: Peck et al (2002)

Against this background, debate continues about exactly what these findings mean in practice. With both positives and negatives (as well as the problem of attribution), the study raised important questions about the extent to which structural change is the best way of achieving more effective partnership (see also below for further discussion):

> The establishment of the combined Trust did not – at the conclusion of the evaluation period – appear to have delivered significant benefits that have not been delivered elsewhere in England without the transfer of social care staff to NHS employment. There is no way of knowing whether comparable changes would have been achieved in Somerset without the creation of the combined Trust.... Further, this is not to say that other, and perhaps more profound, changes will not follow, especially as Somerset has already put in place the transfer of employment of most social care staff

—

> that other localities may have to undertake in time. (Peck
> et al, 2002, p 41)

Equally, the concerns of service users about staff attitudes and about acute care do not appear to have been resolved by the creation of the Partnership Trust. Disappointing though this may be, in one sense it should hardly be surprising. If tackling these concerns was really the main priority, then arguably a different approach would have been more appropriate. Indeed, it is even possible that the integration of health and social care focused management attention so much on the *process* of partnership working that there was less emphasis on user priorities, at least in the short term.

However, perhaps the main complexity of the Somerset study is in trying to understand the overall messages that it tells us about health and social care partnerships:

- According to one reading of the Somerset story, the integration of health and social care achieved nothing that could not have been achieved with a lesser form of partnership working and less upheaval – despite all the changes, nothing essentially seemed to change for service users. If this is the case, the argument goes, it must surely raise major concerns about whether such integration is really worth the effort.
- On the other hand, other commentators look at Somerset and say that local leaders were able to pioneer new ways of working across agency boundaries and to create a new, integrated organisation – all without making anything worse for service users in the meantime. This may then have laid foundations for the future delivery of better outcomes (and we will probably now never know as a result of more recent changes in the area and in mental health services more generally, which mean that is hard to know what, if any, changes to attribute to the integration per se).

Thus, depending on your time frame and on your perspective, Somerset was either a major success or a major storm in a tea cup, and the extent to which partnership working really might achieve better outcomes for people who use services remains just as much a matter of faith. What is apparent, however, is that structural change can lead to potentially unintended negative outcomes in the short term, and this makes it even more important that health and social care services are clear about what they are trying to achieve and why the inevitable upheaval of organisational change is worth it in the longer run. As the lead evaluator of Somerset often says, 'success often looks like failure part way through. The problem with this is that so does failure' (personal communication). As Chapter 4 discusses, this makes the need to be clear about desired outcomes (and about the best structures and processes to achieve these ends) even more fundamental. This is even more the case since subsequent reorganisations can make it difficult to say what impacts such changes may have over time, so a local sense of what we're trying to achieve and why this is the best way forward feels crucial.

Torbay (Thistlethwaite, 2011; Farnsworth, 2012)

Following on from the pioneering work of areas such as Somerset, Peter Thistlethwaite's account of Torbay Care Trust provides a fascinating and important contribution to the literature. A key strength is that the author, a former social services senior manager and editor of the UK *Journal of Integrated Care*, was a key player locally, acting as a critical friend to the Care Trust and supporting ongoing evaluation. Thistlethwaite's description is thus more of a story than it is a formal evaluation, setting out how the Care Trust came about, what problems it was meant to solve, how local leaders tried to implement new ways of working, the key barriers and success factors, outcomes achieved and possible next steps. Although Torbay has some unique features (which may mean that the approach adopted here might not necessarily work in other areas), the paper finishes with a series of practical lessons learned which may be crucial to other areas pondering future integration (see Box 2.4). An additional account by the former chief executive also explores what the 2012 Health and Social Care Act may mean for integrated organisations such as Torbay Care Trust, and thus offers an important personal insight into the impact (and sometimes the unintended consequences) of recent policy changes (Farnsworth, 2012). A broader study by Miller et al (2011) looks at the mixed impact of Care Trusts more generally, and so puts the Torbay story in a broader context.

Box 2.4: Lessons from Torbay

- Base any strategy on the benefits being sought for service users/ patients. Specify the benefits in advance, communicate them constantly, invest in the things that will help achieve them, monitor progress, listen to staff experiences, share results and encourage further improvement....
- Establish joint governance early (NHS, local authority and primary care).
- Invest in a professional approach to organisational development/ change management over an appropriate period of time. Cultural, political and organisational differences and financial and other risks do not have to be deal breakers – they can be overcome....
- Make sure senior/middle managers and clinical leaders are engaged from the start and avoid separate management arrangements for individual professions, including social care. Be confident that individual professional practitioners will enjoy opportunities to work more closely with other professionals. Locating teams together will enhance this....
- Make sure everyone understands what is meant by the term 'integration'....

In its entirety, the Torbay approach may not travel well: Torbay is a small and compact community, with its own environment and history.... However, people in Torbay examined evidence from elsewhere, appraised their own performance, built communication and teamwork between stakeholders, made choices, managed risks and reaped rewards: these things are replicable. There is no textbook to guide the process because

---

> local context (especially the interplay of people, relationships and processes) is a key variable. Anyone embarking on this approach needs to conceive of it as a learning process.
> *Source:* Thistlethwaite (2011, pp 23-4)

Integrated care pilots (RAND Europe/Ernst & Young, 2012)

Alongside specific studies in localities such as Somerset and Torbay, the DH's integrated care pilots shed light on attempts to develop more joined-up approaches in 16 different areas of the country. Focusing on different user groups and seeking to integrate in different kinds of ways, the two-year pilots were evaluated by RAND Europe/Ernst & Young (2012) and the results published (at a time when the topic of integrated care was high on the policy agenda). Unfortunately, the overall results were under-whelming, and the research team concluded that (p i):

> Integrated care led to process improvements such as an increase in the use of care plans and the development of new roles for care staff. Staff believed that these process improvements were leading to improvements in care, even if some of the improvements were not yet apparent. A range of other improvements in care were reported by pilots following local evaluations. We have reported these but they lie beyond the scope of the national evaluation.
>
> Patients did not, in general, share the sense of improvement. This could have been because the process changes reflected the priorities and values of staff (a so-called professionalisation of services); because the benefits had not yet become apparent to service users ("too early to tell"); because of poor implementation; or because the interventions were an ineffective way to improve patient experience. We believe that the lack of improvement in patient experience was in part due to professional rather than user-driven change, partly because it was too early to identify impact within the

timescale of the pilots, and partly because, despite having project management skills and effective leadership, some pilots found the complex changes they set for themselves were harder to deliver than anticipated....

A key aim of many pilots was to reduce hospital utilisation. We found no evidence of a general reduction in emergency admissions, but there were reductions in planned admissions and in outpatient attendance.

While there were some improvements in local processes, this did not seem sufficient to significantly improve patient experience or outcomes. Although approaches such as case management might reduce some hospital costs in the long term, there was little evidence that integrated care inevitably reduces costs more generally (and certainly not in the short term). Overall, the evaluation warned policy makers that (p ii):

The scale and complexity of delivering integrated care activities can easily overwhelm even strong leadership and competent project management. While it may seem obvious in theory that integrating activities should be scaled to match local capacity, this was not always the case in practice. In some cases, enthusiastic local leadership produced expectations that were difficult to realise in practice. Changes to practice often took much longer to achieve than anticipated.

The focus on the needs and preferences of end users can easily be lost in the challenging task of building the organisational platform for integration and in organising new methods of delivering professional care. Using performance metrics focused on the end user and strengthening the user voice in the platform for integration might avoid this.

When developing integrating activities there is no one approach that suits all occasions, and local circumstances and path dependencies will be crucial in shaping the pace and direction of change. Integration is not a matter of following pre-given steps or a particular model of delivery, but often involves finding multiple creative ways of reorganising work in new organisational settings to reduce waste and duplication, deliver more preventive care, target resources more effectively or improve the quality of care.

At the time of writing, a series of integrated care 'pioneers' are being identified (DH, 2013), and it remains to be seen whether these will produce different outcomes or not.

What helps and what hinders?

Although the evidence on outcomes is limited, there is a growing body of literature on what partnerships themselves and other local stakeholders feel help in developing interagency relationships. Typically, this literature is much stronger on the pre-existing conditions for a successful partnership and on the factors that should exist in an ideal scenario than it is on what to do if this is not the case in your area. Put simply, there is a slightly simplistic tendency to assume that issues such as trust and reciprocity are fundamental, without necessarily exploring how best to proceed if partner agencies in your area cannot stand each other and never speak!

This overly optimistic element of the literature aside, much of the existing evidence – both from formal research and from practical experience of working in interagency settings – tends to be summarised in a series of frameworks. Often very accessible and succinct, these run the risk of trying to reduce a much more complex reality down into a series of simple 'rules', but do provide a helpful checklist against which to compare current relationships. Two prominent examples are set out in Boxes 2.5 and 2.6, and frontline practitioners and/or managers may wish to follow these up in more detail with a view to using them to understand their own local partnerships in more depth (for a further example, see also Markwell et al, 2003).

—

Although such frameworks are inevitably simple in their approach, they offer a useful shorthand way of trying to understand what helps and what hinders effective partnership working. When used as the authors intended, moreover, they become more of a way of assessing current relationships, understanding what it is possible to achieve in the current context and identifying areas that require further work. At their best, therefore, such tools can help to make sense of the barriers that frontline partnerships experience, as well as offering potential insight into what needs to happen next and cautioning of the need to keep our partnership aspirations realistic.

Box 2.5: The Partnership Assessment Tool

Developed through ongoing research by the former Nuffield Institute at the University of Leeds, the Partnership Assessment Tool (PAT) provides an opportunity for a routine 'health check' of local partnerships, helps to identify areas of potential conflict and provides a developmental framework for establishing a healthy and effective partnership.

Based on six partnership principles, PAT supports local partners to rate their achievement against various key criteria, providing a quick and easy means of analysing results and identifying issues that require further work. The six key principles that PAT explores are the extent to which partners:

- recognise and accept the need for partnership
- develop clarity and realism of purpose
- ensure commitment and ownership
- develop and maintain trust
- create clear and robust partnership arrangements
- monitor, measure and learn.

Available online via the Department for Communities and Local Government, PAT is probably the best known and most widely used of such tools (Hardy et al, 2003).

Box 2.6: The Partnership Readiness Framework

Developed by Greig and Poxton (2001), the Partnership Readiness Framework highlights the key building blocks of successful partnership:

- building and agreeing shared values and principles with a vision of how life should be for people who use services;
- agreeing specific policy shifts that the partnership arrangements are designed to achieve;
- being prepared to explore new service options and not be tied too closely to existing services or providers;
- being clear about what aspects of service and activity are inside and outside the boundaries of the partnership arrangements;
- being clear about organisational roles in terms of responsibilities for and relationships between commissioning, purchasing and providing;
- identifying agreed resource pools and putting to one side unresolved historical disagreements;
- ensuring effective leadership, including senior level commitment to the partnership agenda;
- providing sufficient partnership development capacity rather than it being a small and marginalised part of everyone's role;
- developing and sustaining good personal relationships, creating opportunities and incentives for key players to nurture these relationships in order to promote mutual trust.

Limits of structural change

If we still know relatively little about what works when it comes to health and social care partnerships, we have learned some key lessons about what does not work. In particular, there is growing evidence to suggest that structural integration – by itself – is not an effective means of achieving more effective partnerships or better outcomes for the people who use services. While this is discussed in more detail in another book in this series by Edward Peck and Helen Dickinson (*Managing and leading in inter-agency settings*), the literature on structural

—

change and reorganisation (see, for example, Craig and Manthorpe, 1999; Fulop et al, 2002, 2005; Field and Peck, 2003; Edwards, 2010) suggests that:

- structural change alone rarely achieves its stated objectives;
- in addition to stated drivers for the merger, there are usually unstated drivers (such as addressing managerial or financial deficits and responding to local or national politics);
- the economic benefits are modest at best, and may be out-weighed by unanticipated direct costs and unintended negative consequences (such as a decline in productivity and morale);
- senior management time is often focused on the process of merger, and this can stall positive service development for at least 18 months (if not longer);
- the after-effects of mergers can continue for many years after the change has taken place.

Nor are outcomes necessarily better in the commercial sector. As Field and Peck (2003, p 743) have demonstrated, 'one of the key messages in the literature on [private sector] mergers is that they have happened at an astonishing pace despite the fact that they do not appear to be beneficial when judged on economic criteria'. According to one source, for instance, 54% of acquisitions were regarded as failures (Coopers & Lybrand, 1993). Consequently, many commercial organisations considering mergers have increasingly begun to pay attention to the human (cultural) factors involved in this process, rather than simply trying to create better results by changing structures.

Despite the overwhelming evidence about the limits of structural change, this remains a common approach in public services (particularly in the NHS). As Walshe (2003) has demonstrated, the NHS has been reorganised on an almost constant basis for decades, with four main impacts:

- The proposed benefits of each reform are never achieved in practice, as the system has always been reorganised again before any meaningful evaluation can take place.
- Significant resources (both financial and human) are wasted (through the diversion of senior management time, new offices, new letterheads, new signs etc).
- The process of reform is commonly circular, with similar structures and solutions re-emerging over time.
- Constant change ironically makes the system highly change-resistant, as staff become increasingly cynical and short-term in their focus.

The overall result, as Walshe suggests in a vivid and depressingly accurate summary (2003, p 108), is that the NHS is 'an organizational shantytown in which structures and systems are cobbled together or thrown up hastily in the knowledge that they will be torn down in due course'. At various stages in recent years, of course, structural change has also been put forward as a potential solution to the problematic nature of the health and social care divide, with the Care Trust model (see Glasby and Peck, 2003; Miller et al, 2011) probably the most visible example of this approach. Thus, despite commitments to notions of 'evidence-based policy', the temptation of an apparently quick and bold structural solution seems almost too much to resist, and the risk is that we end up damaging existing health and social care partnerships in the name of trying to support and improve them. At the time of writing, this process shows no sign of abating, with strong emphasis on integrated care, but also a series of massive organisational changes that could easily damage relationships and make joint working harder in the short term.

Of course, the 2012 reforms are a good example of the way in which organisational mergers are often forced on local systems whether or not they are the best way forward in practice. In such situations, staff have no choice but to make the new organisation work as well as it possibly can, and Box 2.7 summarises some of the key messages from the literature on managing and leading during periods of merger and structural change for those agencies that are experiencing such upheavals.

—

Box 2.7: Lessons from the literature on managing organisations during structural change

There are four distinct time periods within the merger process, with different approaches and management behaviour required in each different phase:

Prior to merger, it is important to assess the culture of each of the merging organisations and to use this knowledge as part of a careful strategy for highlighting and recognising the differences between the organisations.

Having decided to merge, managers and leaders should communicate a vision that sets out the purpose of changes and do this in an open and participatory manner.

During merger, key practical steps include providing practical and emotional support for staff, making human resources (HR) the main issue, communicating relentlessly, setting up clear transitional structures to guide and implement the merger, and helping staff to understand the implications of change.

After merger, it is important to monitor and evaluate the impact of the change for at least three years – both in relation to the original objectives and using other measures such as staff attitudes and service user/carer satisfaction.

Source: Dickinson et al (2006)

Whose fault is this lack of evidence?

As a postscript to this chapter, it is important to think through whose fault this situation may be. Is it the politicians (who might be accused of developing policy in advance of the evidence and jumping on the bandwagon of partnership/integrated care)? Is it academics (who have arguably been slow to respond to the partnership agenda)? Is it frontline services (who have perhaps understandably tended to focus more on implementing change than on evaluating its longer-term impact)? In one sense, the answer is probably that all these groups and factors have contributed to our lack of knowledge about the impact of partnership working. And yet, there is probably a fourth culprit as well – the nature of 'evidence' itself.

Although this may sound strange initially, traditional notions of 'evidence-based practice' have often been dominated by formal research and, in health and social care, by approaches associated with medicine and with science (that is, by quantitative research and by very formal and precise methods known as randomised controlled trials and systematic reviews). As a result, current debates about 'the evidence' often tend to focus only on very selective understandings of what should constitute valid evidence, and a large number of dissenting voices are often overlooked. While this is discussed in more detail elsewhere (see, for example, Rycroft-Malone et al, 2004; Glasby and Beresford, 2006; Glasby et al, 2007; Glasby, 2012b), a good example of this is the systematic reviews common in some parts of the NHS, which initially identify several thousand studies, exclude all but a very small number of quantitative studies, then conclude that there is very little research available!

Although clearly a caricature of a much more complex issue, there do seem to be clear instances in both health and social care where a narrow focus on traditional notions of what constitutes valid evidence can lead to a limited insight into the issues at stake (and the issue of health and social care partnerships may well be an example of this). As a result, it is possible that we may understand more about the nature and impact of partnerships if we adopt a different approach to understanding 'what works'. While this is a broader issue than can be dealt with in full here, possible examples include:

• Focusing not on 'what works' so much as on 'what does not work'. While we still know relatively little about the outcomes of partnership working, there is significant evidence of the limitations of single agency approaches. Instead of waiting for 'the evidence' before implementing new ways of working, therefore, an important step forward would be to decide what does not work in the current system, do something different and test out whether this works better (essentially a form of learning 'what works' by doing and reflecting). Inevitably, this might mean a very different role for those national bodies currently responsible for improving health and social care services and for disseminating good practice.

- Basing future decisions not just on what formal research has to tell us, but also on what we believe we have learned from previous changes and from current ways of working (essentially a move away from 'evidence-based practice' to a notion of 'practice-based evidence').
- Expanding traditional (often very medically dominated) notions of evidence to include other ways of knowing the world, such as the lived experience of users and carers, and the tacit knowledge of frontline practitioners (essentially a move away from traditional 'evidence-based practice' to a broader, more inclusive notion of 'knowledge-based practice').

Thus, the overall result of this discussion is that we do not yet know what impact partnership working has, for whom or under what circumstances. However, the reality is that we are probably unlikely to know this with any certainty for some time (if ever). As a result, the best way forward in the short term may be for health and social care practitioners and their organisations to be clear about what they are trying to achieve by working together, and to build in appropriate critical reflection and evaluation to enable them to learn as they go along. (In many ways, this builds on a broader theoretical approach known as 'realistic evaluation', and Chapter 4 provides a more detailed summary of the key concepts and frameworks that this entails.) While such an approach may not always seem very convincing to a busy manager or a national policy maker under pressure to ensure that their next policy is 'evidence-based', this nevertheless seems a more constructive way forward than arguing that we cannot do anything because we do not have enough 'evidence'.

—

Reflective exercises

1. With a colleague from a different professional or organisational background, what outcomes have you been able to achieve together that you couldn't have achieved by yourself? Are these outcomes for people using services, for your organisation, for colleagues, or a combination? What helped and hindered your attempts to work together?
2. Think of a local partnership or service trying to deliver integrated care. Using the frameworks in Boxes 2.5 and 2.6, how well do local partners seem to be working together and where could they improve?
3. After reading the health and social care trade press, pick a recent example of a policy or service trying to deliver more integrated care. What would success look like for this policy/service, and how would you go about evaluating it?
4. Look at some of the formal evaluations in 'Further reading and resources' below. What types of evidence have they collected and how clear-cut/easy to interpret are their findings? If you were a minister or a local leader receiving such a study, what would you do with it in practical terms?

Further reading and resources

For key studies, see the national evaluations of partnership initiatives, such as:

- The Children's Fund (Edwards et al, 2006)
- Children's trusts (University of East Anglia, 2007)
- The Health Act flexibilities (Glendinning et al, 2002b)
- HAZs (Barnes et al, 2005)
- Intermediate care (Godfrey et al, 2005; Barton et al, 2006)
- Sure Start (Belsky et al, 2007)
- DH integrated care pilots (RAND Europe/Ernst & Young, 2012)

—

At a more local level, a particularly important insight is provided by Peck et al's (2002) innovative study of health and social care partnerships in Somerset and a discussion of the Torbay experience by Thistlethwaite (2011) and Farnsworth (2012). At a national level, the RAND/Ernst & Young (2012) study of the government's integrated care pilots provides a key overview, while Glasby and Dickinson's (2009) edited text, *International perspectives on health and social care*, places the UK experience in a broader, international context. For summaries of the literature, see key reviews by Cameron and Lart (2003), Dowling et al (2004), Perkins et al (2010) and Cameron et al (2012). For a critical and more theoretical summary of the limitations of current approaches to evaluating partnerships, see Helen Dickinson's book in this series, *Evaluating outcomes in health and social care*.

3

Hot topics and emerging issues

Having explored key concepts and summarised key research findings, this chapter explores a series of current tensions in the relationship between health, social care and other partners, including:

- Can effective partnerships ever be 'forced' by central policy?
- How do we ensure accountability, and what happens when money is involved?
- How can we be responsible for services delegated to partner agencies?
- How do we ensure that partnerships remain focused on what service users and patients want?
- What are the implications of clinical commissioning?
- Do partnerships lead to better outcomes, and what impact will the current financial climate have?

Sadly, with the lack of evidence described in Chapter 2, it is hard to be definitive about many (if any) of these questions. In many ways, therefore, the issues explored below represent a good example of areas in which lessons learned the hard way in frontline policy and practice are far ahead of the evidence from formal research. However, the discussion below is an attempt to draw together – from various sources – what we already know about such 'hot topics', and to pose a series of additional challenges for frontline practitioners and services seeking to develop more effective partnerships to reflect on.

Legal duties and 'forced' partnerships

While much of the literature on effective partnership working emphasises issues such as trust, reciprocity, autonomy and shared vision, there are many examples of situations in which partners have no choice but to work in partnership. At a national level, statutes such as the 1999/2006 Health Act, the 2004 Children Act, the 2007 Local Government and Public Involvement in Health Act and the 2012 Health and Social Care Act set out various duties to cooperate, to work in partnership and to promote more integrated care. However, such commitments are often very vague, and are typically more symbolic than practical when it comes to ensuring effective partnerships at a local level. Although it is a slightly tongue-in-cheek example, what would happen to a health and social care community that was deemed to be breaking its statutory obligations to work in partnership? How would we identify such a breach of the law, prove the accusation and hold the agencies concerned to account? In any case, what do such duties actually mean in practice, and at what stage in a problematic relationship do we decide that such legal duties are not being discharged? Even if all these questions were answered, what would happen in practice to the chief executives of each partner agency? As some policy commentators suggest in private, when the first fine is levied or the first senior manager 'named and shamed' for failure to collaborate across agency boundaries, then such legal duties may be perceived as having more 'teeth' than at present (personal communications).

In practice, of course, such legal provisions send out a potentially powerful symbolic message about the importance that policy makers attach to partnership working – by devising duties of partnership, those who make our laws are effectively sending a very clear and welcome signal that not working together is not an option and will not be tolerated. However, moving from a general symbolic message such as this to implementing and supporting lasting change is a more complex and fraught process. While these issues are discussed in much more detail in the broader literature on policy making (see, for example, Hill, 2004; Buse et al, 2005; Baggott, 2007), recent partnership policies have been designed in very different ways with very different underlying assumptions about what motivates frontline practitioners and about what changes behaviour at ground level.

—

At its most extreme, this debate often focuses on the extent to which it is either possible or desirable to compel practitioners and local organisations to work together (for a discussion of so-called *mandated collaboration*, see Rodríguez et al, 2007). A good example of this issue is the debate around how best to reduce the number of people whose stay in hospital is delayed due to problems in the discharge process. While hospital discharge has long been a problematic area of policy and practice (for a summary, see Glasby, 2003), it became an increasing policy priority from 2000 onwards following government concerns that delays attributed to social care may be jeopardising commitments around NHS waiting times. Following the investment of additional money, the main response from policy makers in England was the controversial 2003 Community Care (Delayed Discharges etc) Act, which introduced a system of 'cross-charging' (subsequently described as a system of 'reimbursement'). From the beginning, such a policy divided commentators. While some felt that this was an overly simplistic approach that unfairly penalised social care for what was essentially an interagency issue, others claimed that delaying hospital discharge due to delays in arranging or funding social care services was unacceptable and had to be tackled. In particular, much of the discussion centred on the extent to which such an apparently punitive approach was the best way of promoting the long-term interagency relationships required to tackle the root of the problem (see Box 3.1).

Box 3.1: Reimbursement and hospital discharge as an example of 'forced' partnership

As Henwood (2006) explains, the 2003 Community Care (Delayed Discharges etc) Act introduced a system whereby NHS bodies must notify social services of a patient's likely need for community care services (a Section 2 notification). There is a defined timescale (at least three days) for social services to complete the individual's assessment and to provide appropriate social care services. A second notice (a Section 5 notification) follows completion of a multidisciplinary assessment, and gives notice of the proposed day of discharge (minimum of 24 hours notice). A reimbursement charge of £100 per day (£120 per day in London/the South East) is paid by social services to the acute trust if the fact of social services not having met their obligations is the sole reason for the delay in discharge from hospital. NHS bodies have to make both of the notifications to social services if a claim for reimbursement is to be triggered. Liability for payment begins on the day after the three days of the assessment notification, or the day after the proposed discharge date, whichever is later.

As soon as this policy was announced, there were immediate concerns that this would encourage premature discharge and emergency readmission, that it would damage existing relationships between health and social care and that it unfairly penalised one partner for a genuinely whole systems problem. In contrast, others argued that hospital was an inappropriate place for older people in particular to be when they no longer needed the services provided there, and that any policy that encouraged swift discharge and a more effective use of scarce resources was to be welcomed.

Following the implementation of the new system, delays did initially fall (although they had already been falling before the new policy and the rate of reduction then levelled off before sometimes creeping back up). In the main, health and social care communities have typically worked hard to ensure that the 'horror stories' predicted by some commentators have not materialised, and many have negotiated a system whereby both partners invest in rehabilitative services, with no charges payable until the level of the 'fines' amassed exceeds the amount that social care has invested up-front in new services. However, concerns remain that such a policy may not be the best way of securing long-term change and that the introduction of such financial incentives may have unintended consequences (for example, on the risk of premature discharge, on the rate of care home admissions from hospital and/or on the rate of emergency hospital readmissions).

For further discussion, see CSCI (2004, 2005), Glasby (2003), Henwood (2004, 2006), Godfrey et al (2008) and McCoy et al (2007).

In an important contribution to this debate, Rodríguez et al (2007) argue that 'mandated collaboration' involves three different types of governance:

- bureaucratic mechanisms (such as the introduction of new rules and regulations);
- new incentives to encourage partners to alter previous behaviour;
- interaction between partners to aid mutual understanding.

Returning to the earlier discussion about different ways of organising public services (see Chapter 1), Rodríguez et al see these approaches as representative of the three organisational types explored in Box 1.2:

- hierarchical approaches to compel joint working;
- market-based approaches to provide new incentives;
- network-based approaches to enable more informal interaction, shared values and cooperation.

According to this analysis, many attempts at 'forced partnership' may fail if they concentrate solely on mandating the partnership, without sufficient rules, incentives or interaction to make the policy work. Applying this to the discussion of reimbursement above, initial policy certainly seems to have been guilty of this approach, with subsequent attempts to implement the policy enjoying more success as a result of a more nuanced blend of hierarchy, market and network (for a discussion of the need for 'requisite variety', see also Peck and 6, 2006).

Of course, the extent to which it is possible to create 'forced' partnerships is actually an outward manifestation of a deeper issue: how best to encourage change in public services. Again, this is discussed in more detail in the policy literature. However, our own belief is that previous policies have attempted to change behaviour at the front line in at least three different ways:

- by 'making' people behave differently (through the use of legislation or mechanisms such as reimbursement above);

- by the 'power of ideas' (exhorting people to behave differently and appealing to rational debate about the best way forward);
- by 'structural change' (see Chapter 2 for a critique of our tendency to rely on this approach in the NHS in particular).

For any given social issue and policy response, a mix of these approaches may be required in practice (and the nature of that balance will change according to the current context, the nature of the issue and the perceived urgency of the issues at stake). However, we believe that a more powerful way of changing practice is to *change accountabilities*, and that the other approaches summarised above often get used in the short term only as a more superficial and simplistic proxy. It is for this reason, we would argue, that repeated NHS reorganisation seems to have little effect (although this looks like and is often justified in terms of changing accountabilities, it typically happens so frequently and focuses so much on structural change that the underlying accountabilities remain the same). It is also for this reason that social care policies such as direct payments and individual budgets seem so exciting and potentially transformative (as they fundamentally alter the accountability between services and welfare professionals on the one hand, and people who use services on the other; for an introduction to direct payments, see Glasby and Littlechild, 2009).

Accountability and risk

In Chapter 1, we suggested that partnership working has traditionally been seen as a 'good thing', but that there has been more recent recognition of some of the negatives associated with partnerships. In many ways, this is part of a more recent reaction against partnerships, in which frontline services and practitioners are (perhaps rightly) starting to adopt what we see as a more sceptical approach. In many ways this trend is illustrated by growing concerns about issues of risk and accountability, and by a 2005 report published by the Audit Commission, *Governing partnerships*. According to the latter, partnerships can be crucial in delivering improvements in people's quality of life, but

—

can also bring risks as well as opportunities. In particular, partnerships may not always deliver value for money (given the direct and indirect costs associated), while the complexity and ambiguity that partnership working entails can 'generate confusion and weaken accountability' (p 2). In addition, the Commission found that areas such as leadership, decision making, scrutiny and risk management were all under-developed in partnerships. Above all, 'local public bodies should be much more constructively critical about this form of working: it may not be the best solution in every case' (Audit Commission, 2005, p 2).

While these issues are discussed in more detail by Glasby and Peck (2006) and in the book on leadership in this series (*Managing and leading in inter-agency settings*, by Edward Peck and Helen Dickinson), current and recent partnerships do seem increasingly concerned to be clear about their accountabilities and about what happens when money is involved. In many ways, this is entirely right and proper, and no one would presumably argue against greater transparency about such important issues. However, quite how to achieve this in practice remains problematic, and opinions vary as to the best way forward. While the Audit Commission (2005) emphasises the need for 'partnership agreements' as a means of ensuring good governance, we have a slightly different take on the issues (for a more detailed analysis, see Glasby and Peck, 2006). According to our earlier discussion about hierarchies, markets and networks (see Chapter 1), some would argue that a crucial feature of partnerships is the extent to which they enable individual organisations to retain the right of exit (which is very different to a market-based contract, for example). Playing devil's advocate somewhat, any partners that need very detailed legal agreement about respective roles and responsibilities would surely be better off signing a formal contract rather than opting for the more informal and flexible approach that a partnership entails. Presumably for some partners it is exactly this flexibility and this right of exit that makes partnership an attractive proposition in the first place, and subsequent governance arrangements need to strike an appropriate balance between protection, probity, room for manoeuvre and clarity of roles and responsibilities. As a very rough rule of thumb (and only

—

slightly tongue in cheek), it has been suggested that any partnership that needs an agreement that is more than a few pages long is probably not really a partnership in the first place.

Working through partner agencies

Closely linked to issues of risk and accountability is a further question about how best to ensure that individual agencies continue to meet their moral and legal obligations once they have delegated day-to-day responsibility for delivering services to a partner agency. It was precisely this issue that lay at the heart of the formal investigation in Cornwall, with inspectors (Healthcare Commission/CSCI, 2006, p 7) arguing that services delivered via a so-called NHS 'partnership' trust had very little involvement from social care at all and that relationships between the trust and the county council were poor (for a summary of some of the key partnership-related findings, see Box 3.2).

Box 3.2: Findings from an investigation into services for people with learning difficulties

In 2006, a joint investigation into the provision of services for people with learning difficulties at Cornwall Partnership NHS Trust found evidence of institutional abuse, poor practice and a lack of appropriate leadership (Healthcare Commission/CSCI, 2006, p 7). In addition, inspectors found that:

- PCT commissioning of services was inadequate, with insufficient monitoring.
- 'Working relationships between the Trust and Cornwall County Council have been poor for a considerable time.'
- 'Services for people with learning disabilities were not transferred to social services, following the closure of long stay hospitals, as they were in other parts of the UK.'
- 'Social services have had little involvement in the care provided by the Trust.'

- Learning disability services were marginalised, both within the Trust itself (which focused primarily on mental health services) and by the Strategic Health Authority.

Ironically, inpatient services for people with learning difficulties have since been the focus of national concerns following a high profile Panorama programme and a subsequent national programme of inspections (see CQC, 2012). Reading these stories, it is hard to avoid the conclusion that some patients can enter services where they are 'out of sight and out of mind', and that this might make it difficult for partners that have delegated a particular service or responsibility to another to stay fully engaged on an ongoing basis.

Responding to this dilemma is difficult, and many organisations find it hard to get the balance right between giving a lead partner the flexibility to deliver on joint priorities while at the same time remaining sufficiently involved to be able both to support and to scrutinise that partner. All too often, this seems to result in a situation where the original partner either delegates formal responsibilities (yet does not really trust the other partner to deliver), or sees any functions it has delegated as 'somebody else's problem' and actively disengages. Certainly, this seemed to be a potential risk with the creation of Care Trusts, with some health organisations finding it difficult to retain a strong relationship with their local council once powers had been delegated to the NHS (Miller et al, 2011). To guard against these dangers, new Health and Well-being Boards *may* offer a forum in which partners can take a step back and look at the whole health and local government system in the round, but there is no guarantee that this is a role they will feel comfortable with or find easy in practice.

Staying focused on service users

Part of the problem with the current policy context is that partnerships are now so widespread that it is hard to continue to see them as a means to an end. This is a consistent theme throughout this book, and is explored in more detail in Chapter 4. However, opinion is divided as to whether partnership working is a 'good thing' from the perspective of people who use services. While some claim that partnerships are a potentially helpful way of responding to the needs of service users and to their desire for more integrated care, others see greater partnership working as leading to reduced choice and a greater concentration of power in favour of services rather than of service users. A good example here is provided by debates in mental health services, with some commentators arguing that the integration of health and social care runs the risk of denying service users access to more social, non-medical alternatives to traditional psychiatric approaches (see Box 3.3). Similarly, greater collaboration between services such as health and social care offers the potential of more coordinated, better resourced and more meaningful approaches to user and patient involvement, while at the same time running the risk of reducing sources of support and opportunities to voice their concerns should service users be dissatisfied with current services.

Box 3.3: Ambiguities of partnership working from a user perspective: the case of mental health services

Potential advantages of partnership (in theory):

- single point of entry
- less sense of being passed 'from pillar to post'
- more holistic response to need
- greater coordination of support
- broader range of services.

Potential disadvantages:

- scope for medical model to dominate other perspectives
- potential for more social alternatives to be overshadowed by psychiatric approaches

- less chance for one partner to advocate on behalf of users with the other partner
- possible loss of local services as the partnership rationalises its provision
- having one point of contact can give users nowhere else to go if this attempt to contact services does not work as well as it should
- concerns about a loss of key relationships with staff and about potential change in use of local buildings.

Source: Personal communications, service users receiving support from Partnership Trusts

In addition to these issues, Skelcher et al (2004) raise a series of challenges about the threats that partnerships can pose to local democracy. In a series of research studies and commentaries, they argue that partnerships can be a flexible vehicle by which entrepreneurial managers exercise greater discretion over local services and that partnerships often engage the public and service users in their work. However, decision makers on partnership boards are typically public service managers, and the subsequent partnership can bypass traditional forms of local democracy and accountability (that is, elected members and local councils). Partnerships also have very different and variable approaches to issues such as public access, transparency and openness, with standards typically falling below accepted good practice. As part of this debate, Skelcher et al (2004) have developed a Governance Assessment Tool (see Box 3.4) that partnerships can use to assess the extent to which they conform to current good practice standards around such issues of accountability and probity.

Box 3.4: Governance Assessment Tool

Public accessibility

1. Are meetings of the board advertised?
2. Are meetings of the board open to the press and public?
3. Are the public entitled to see reports considered by the board?
4. Are the reports that the board will consider available for the public to consult prior to the meeting?
5. Are the public entitled to see minutes of board meetings?
6. Is there an annual general meeting that the public can attend?

Internal governance

1. Does the partnership have a memorandum of association or other document defining its role and powers?
2. Does the partnership have a written constitution or set of standing orders defining how it will conduct its business at meetings?
3. Is membership for a limited period of time? If so, for how long?
4. Does a quorum apply at board meetings? If so, what is it?
5. Are written minutes of board meetings produced?
6. Are there allowances or other payments for members? If so, how much?

Member conduct

1. Is there a code of conduct to regulate the behaviour of members at board meetings?
2. If there is a code, are board members required to agree to be bound by it?
3. Is there a register in which board members detail their financial and other interests? If so, is this compulsory? And is it open for public inspection?

4. Is there a system for declaring conflicts of interest at meetings? If so, what is the procedure and where is it set down?
5. Is there a procedure for ensuring that members declaring conflicts of interest take no part in the decision? If so, what is the procedure and where is it set down?

Accountability

1. Does the partnership have to prepare an annual report? If yes, is this a public document?
2. Does the partnership have to prepare an annual budget? If yes, is this a public document?
3. Does the partnership have to prepare annual accounts? If yes, is this a public document?
4. Is the partnership subject to external audit?
5. Is the partnership subject to external inspection?
6. Is there a complaints process available to citizens or service users?
7. Is the partnership under the jurisdiction of an ombudsman or inspectorate?
8. Is the partnership required to meet targets agreed with any other bodies?
9. Does the partnership make a formal report to any other bodies (including the member organisations)?
10. Can members be recalled by their nominating bodies?

Source: Skelcher et al (2004)

Helpful though this tool is as a means of thinking through governance issues, it does tend to assume that current approaches in local government represent a gold standard against which other ways of delivering services should be judged. While this may be true in terms of the formal rules that govern conduct and access in local government, the reality is arguably a system in which such theoretical rights become less meaningful as a result of difficulties that many members of the public face when seeking to understand and engage with the culture and bureaucracy of many local authorities. Although the NHS is often portrayed as having a 'democratic deficit', a more accurate description would be to say that social care is accountable to locally elected politicians, while the NHS is accountable nationally to a Secretary of State who is appointed by the democratically elected government of the day. With low turnouts in recent local elections, moreover, it is at least debatable as to whether the Secretary of State or the local councillor has a greater democratic mandate.

Ultimately, therefore, what is at stake here may be two alternative visions of the future:

- Will two already large, powerful and frequently inaccessible public services combine to become even larger, even more powerful and even more inaccessible?
- Or will greater partnership working prompt current organisations and professions to be more responsive to the needs and desires of service users, help them to reflect on the strengths and limitations of what they currently do, and enable them to challenge established practice where it does not function in the best interests of people who use services?

Clinical commissioning

In England, the 2012 Health and Social Care Act abolished previous PCTs and Strategic Health Authorities, introducing a new national NHS Commissioning Board (NHS England), new Commissioning Support Services and new Clinical Commissioning Groups (CCGs). While this legislation proved highly controversial (for a fascinating overview, see Timmins, 2012), the reforms essentially make primary care responsible for commissioning local health services on behalf of the whole population. Although this has many similarities with previous forms of primary care-led commissioning, it nevertheless shifts GPs from a role as the champion of the individual patient into one of being responsible for the needs of the whole population (and for making potentially difficult decisions about which services should be provided and how to make best use of increasingly scarce public resources). GPs will then come together with local councillors and other key stakeholders via new Health and Well-being Boards.

Quite what this means for joint working remains to be seen. In many ways, GPs feel like the 'forgotten partners' of previous reforms, with the emphasis tending to be on the broader relationship between the local authority and former PCTs. In many areas, there was a flurry of joint activity in the late 1990s, with a series of GP-attached social work pilots and with social services representatives sitting on the boards of new Primary Care Groups (PCGs). However, the advent of PCTs tended to shift the focus away from relationships in general practice, and many social workers and GPs have little contact with each other or knowledge of each other's roles.

Despite these changes, the broader literature suggests that relationships with general practice have been difficult and under-developed over time. Thus, a key text from 1981 stresses that:

> From the late 1940s closer collaboration between social work and general medical practice has been advocated as a means of improving primary health care. Despite the persuasive rhetoric of its advocates and the successful completion of several demonstration projects of attachment of social workers to group medical practices, the majority of general practitioners and social workers in the field remain unconvinced, not so much of the potential but of the possibility of inter-occupational collaboration. (Huntingdon, 1981, p 1)

More recently, a review of relationships in older people's services suggests that:

> British GPs have ... historically been independent contractors, and until very recently remained largely outside mainstream NHS organisations and management structures....The history of GPs' collaborative activities, either with one another

or with social services, is not promising.... GPs were not involved in the joint health and social services planning and commissioning that took place from the 1970s, and when they did become involved, during the quasi-market of the 1990s, it was as GP fund-holders, who used their enhanced financial flexibility and purchasing leverage to buy additional social work services for their practices and their patients.... Even among leading-edge GP fund-holders, engagement with wider strategic planning and inter-agency activities was minimal.... Moreover, inter-professional relationships between doctors and social workers have been regarded by both academics and professionals themselves as poor, being characterised by a lack of mutual understanding and blame and therefore providing an unhelpful basis for collaboration. (Glendinning et al, 2002c, p 190)

The result of all this seems to be that the advent of clinical commissioning could offer new opportunities for joint working, but could also jeopardise existing relationships and joint approaches. Elsewhere, we have described this as an opportunity for 'new conversations with old players', but have warned that early and significant attention will be needed to make sure that joint working does not become even harder in the short term as new approaches are bedding in (see Box 3.5 for a summary of recent research).

Box 3.5: New conversations with old players? Joint working between general practice and social care

In 2013, a School for Social Care Research report reviewed the relationship between social care and general practice, building on a previous study by Rummery and Glendinning (2000). This found that:

- Little had been published on this topic since a small number of key local and national evaluations in the late 1990s and early 2000s, and this seems a major gap given the current emphasis on clinical commissioning.

- Some of the literature is very aspirational about the potential of joint working, but is often published in non-peer-reviewed and/or more practice-focused journals. While this material contains helpful summaries of lessons learned, it can also be very descriptive and does not always cite direct evidence for the claims made.
- More rigorous studies with more detailed/transparent methodologies and in peer-reviewed journals tend to cite mixed or under-whelming results, suggesting that joint working by itself is insufficient to produce significantly better outcomes.

Overall, the study concluded that:

> This review of the relationship between social care and primary care raises a series of key issues for future research, policy and practice. In terms of the formal literature, we know relatively little about joint working between social care and general practice, with a limited evidence base (much of it deriving from the early 2000s, from the advent of PCGs and/or from a number of GP-attached social work or integrated team pilots). As with the broader partnership literature, key issues seem to include the practical difficulties of engaging GPs in inter-agency collaborations; a lack of mutual understanding; different priorities and geographical boundaries; and a turbulent policy context. Key factors that may aid more effective joint working include the importance of time and space to build good relationships; trust and awareness of each other's roles; clear commitment at practice and senior level; shared priorities and outcomes; and appropriate practical and organisational development support.

From our interviews, recent changes have created opportunities for new relationships – but the consensus seems to be that this will be challenging for new CCGs and that progress may be difficult in a very complex policy environment. Over time, general practice and social care have had very little direct contact, with previous relationships focusing on the local authority and the PCT. Initial training also does little to prepare either agency/ profession to collaborate, and there are a series of practical barriers to overcome. There is also a need to clarify how key parts of the new system such as Commissioning Support Services [CSSs] and the NHS Commissioning Board will work and link with local bodies. While the former may offer scope for more integrated approaches at local level, the uncertainty surrounding the role of CSSs may also undermine efforts at joint working.

Source: Glasby et al (forthcoming)

Integrated care in a cold climate: do partnerships lead to better outcomes?

Underneath much of the analysis that runs throughout this book are several unanswered questions about the extent to which partnerships or integrated care lead to better outcomes, how we would know if they did and whether the effort involved in developing partnerships is really worth it. While this is examined in more detail by Helen Dickinson's book in the current series, *Evaluating outcomes in health and social care*, Chapters 1 and 2 of this book have started to develop and reiterate two key points:

- the assumption that partnerships lead to better outcomes is at best unproven, and much existing partnership working remains essentially faith-based;

- both policy makers and frontline services need to focus more on the outcomes they are trying to achieve, before considering the structures and the processes they want to develop as a result.

Of course, such issues are even more crucial in an age of austerity than they were in an era of relative plenty. Thus, a key difference between the first and second editions of this book is the context in which partnerships/integrated care are being seen as a potential solution to the problems of the health and social care system. As money gets tighter it may well be that working together is even more important but even harder than ever before, and that the themes covered in this book become even more fundamental. Arguably under New Labour the additional funds that were made available for collaboration meant, to some extent, that joint working remained on the periphery of organisations, reserved for particular projects or certain individuals with boundary spanning roles. The challenge today is therefore to mainstream more joined-up working without additional funding and at a time when many public service organisations are actively cutting budgets. With this in mind, Chapter 4 moves on to provide some conceptual frameworks to help explore these issues in more detail, to help develop more locally appropriate approaches to partnership working/integration, and to focus on ensuring that subsequent interagency relationships are more tailored to local contexts and focused on desired outcomes.

Reflective exercises

1. Think about a successful partnership or an integrated service that is delivering real benefits for service users. How did this come about, and what motivates staff and local services to work in this way? What incentives or sanctions can national policy makers use to encourage more integrated care? Can policy 'make' people work together and if so, how? If it can't, what approaches might be more successful?

2. Reflecting on local services, how do partners balance/share risk and rewards? How do relationships change if money is directly involved? Are appropriate safeguards in place to protect people if something goes wrong (without this getting in the way of doing what's best for service users and cares)?

3. If one partner has delegated responsibilities to another, how can it strike an appropriate balance between staying involved in debates about the service in question while also leaving its partner sufficiently free to do what is needed? Can you think of practical examples where this balance has been about right, and where it has felt wrong?

4. Think of a local partnership and analyse it from different perspectives. Which outcomes is it trying to achieve and who decides? Are outcomes for service users, for staff and for local organisations compatible with each other, or are there tensions between different notions of success?

5. For English readers, what impact might clinical commissioning have on current joint working and relationships?

6. Think about local services and relationships in the area where you live or work. What impact is the broader economic climate having on the extent to which people work together (or not)? Will austerity encourage more integrated care (because we have to work together to respond to the challenges we face) or will it damage existing relationships? Irrespective of the broader economy, what can you do as an individual to contribute to more integrated care?

Further reading and resources

This chapter has covered a broad range of issues, and readers may want to follow up specific topics in more detail. As a result, the further reading and resources below are necessarily diverse to enable people to explore all the issues that are relevant to them and their local context.

For more information on delayed hospital discharge, see sources such as CSCI (2004, 2005), Glasby (2003), Henwood (2004, 2006), Godfrey et al (2008) and McCoy et al (2007).

For material on working with broader partners, see contributions by Benson (1975) and Hudson (2004); see also Box 4.3 for further discussion.

For a discussion of the balance to be struck between effective partnership and local democratic processes, see Skelcher et al's (2004) work on governance and accountability. In particular, their Governance Assessment Tool provides a useful and accessible means of assessing the extent to which partnerships conform to current good practice standards around issues such as accessibility, transparency, accountability and probity.

For examples of what can happen when things go wrong, journalistic accounts of breakdowns in local partnerships can be a helpful resource (see, for example, Batty, 2003; O'Hara, 2006). The Audit Commission (2005) also provides an important discussion of issues of risk, accountability and governance.

An accessible discussion of interagency partnerships and governance – *We have to stop meeting like this* – was written by Glasby and Peck (2006) for the former Integrated Care Network.

Rummery and Glendinning (2000) and Glasby et al (forthcoming) have both produced reviews of the relationship between social care and general practice.

4

Useful frameworks and concepts

So far, previous chapters in this book have tended to problematise the concept of partnership working/integration, to critique current policy and practice, and to provide more questions than answers. In some respects, this chapter is little different in that the issues at stake are so difficult that definitive answers are unlikely. However, with this caveat in mind, this chapter seeks to develop previous discussions by summarising a series of useful theoretical frameworks and approaches to help unpick some of the themes and issues cited earlier.

The importance of outcomes

Above all, this book has stressed the importance of being clear (with each other, with staff and with service users) what outcomes our partnerships are designed to achieve. This has included:

- a critique of the literature for focusing on issues of process (how well are we working together?) rather than on outcomes (does it make any difference for people who use services?);
- a critique of the tendency to assume that partnership working is a 'good thing' (that leads to better services and hence to better outcomes);
- a critique of the tendency to focus on potentially positive outcomes without necessarily considering the negatives of partnership working;
- a critique of traditional notions of evidence-based practice (which have often been too narrow and too focused on particular types of

research methodology to help us fully understand the relationship between partnerships and outcomes);

- a critique of the tendency to see partnership working as an end in itself rather than as a means to an end;
- a critique of a potential lack of clarity about exactly which forms of partnership may be most appropriate to deliver desired outcomes (see below).

In response, a useful approach for guarding against these dangers derives from the broader literature on 'theories of change' and 'realistic evaluation'. While these approaches are described in more detail elsewhere (see, for example, Pawson and Tilley, 1997; Connell and Kubisch, 1998; Dickinson, 2006), Figure 4.1 builds on these insights to set out a simple three-step approach that asks frontline services and practitioners to consider:

- what they are trying to achieve for local people (outcomes)
- how well (or otherwise) current services do this already (context)
- the structures they need to develop as a result (process).

Figure 4.1: Focusing on outcomes

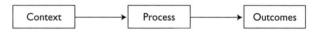

While this is inevitably an over-simplification, thinking of partnership working in these terms can be a helpful way of concentrating on what is important. Depending on the outcomes concerned, local partners may well decide that they do need some form of partnership, but this is not automatically assumed, and the type of relationship required depends on where local services are starting and what they want to achieve. Simple though this may appear, remaining focused on outcomes is extremely difficult, as many policy makers, managers and practitioners tend to find it easier to think in terms of structures and processes rather than outcomes. This seems to be the result of a series of interrelated issues – the historical legacy that current services have inherited, the tendency for performance management systems to focus more on process than on outcomes, and the fact that many frontline practitioners are often never asked to think about what they are there to achieve on behalf of the people they serve. In addition, the process of determining outcomes may not be simple and can reveal that different stakeholders have quite different perceptions about what the partnership does/should do. If such an exercise does indeed reveal significant differences, it may well help to explain why partnership working may have been problematic – because different people had very different expectations of the relationship. However, with all these caveats, the fact remains that such an approach can help potential partners to retain a focus on partnership working/integration as a means to an end, rather than as an end in itself (for an example of what can happen when a focus on outcomes is lost, see Box 4.1).

Against this background, the remainder of this chapter seeks to explore each stage of the diagram in Figure 4.1, summarising some of the key frameworks and concepts that may help to develop our ability to understand issues of outcome, context and process in more detail.

Box 4.1: Remaining focused on outcomes

When asked to focus on outcomes, most public service managers and practitioners quickly drift back into issues of process. If asked, many health and social care communities might articulate desired outcomes in terms of 'a single point of entry', 'quicker access to services' or 'a single assessment'.

Important though all these may be, none are outcomes for service users. On the contrary, all are processes, and further facilitation is often needed to help participants understand what kind of outcomes (fewer admissions to hospital, greater life expectancy, greater satisfaction with services etc) they think these processes may help them achieve.

Although this may seem pedantic, being clear about the difference between the overall outcome and the processes that may help you get there is important – we are so conditioned to think about the world in particular ways that we rarely stop to ask ourselves deeper questions about the best way forward. For example, if we really are trying to reduce hospital admissions, a single assessment and a single point of entry may be the right way forward; equally, if this is genuinely what we are trying to achieve, then we might do something else entirely (which may or may not involve a partnership).

In an informative if depressing example, one health and social care community was adamant that the outcome it was trying to achieve for local older people was an integrated management team. We are yet to meet any older people who need or want an integrated management team from their health and social care services – this is simply a process that may or may not be the best way of trying to achieve different and better outcomes for people who use services.

When seeking to make a clear statement about the outcomes that any given partnership is designed to achieve, recent policy and practice reveals a number of helpful hints. In particular, anecdotal evidence from previous reforms in children's services suggests that this can be most powerful when outcomes are focused on potential benefits for people who use services, when they are expressed positively (that is, 'keeping children safe and well' rather than 'preventing abuse'), and when they are simple and easy to communicate to staff, service users and the public alike. In addition, it is our belief that it is at the stage of articulating desired outcomes that user and carer involvement is most important. All too often, in our experience, services ask users for their views on issues of structure or process. While users may have a view on service structures, we believe that their input is crucial from day one, and that they should be centrally involved in discussions about desired outcomes – what do they want their lives to be like and how can services support this? After this, involvement in critiquing the current context is also important (in order to establish the extent to which current services deliver user aspirations), but involvement in what structures are needed as a result is much more technical and much less relevant to many service users. As an example of such an approach, Box 4.2 summarises the Health Services Management

Centre's Partnership Outcomes Evaluation Toolkit (POETQ) as a possible way of approaching this issue (see also the book by Helen Dickinson in this series for further details: *Evaluating outcomes in health and social care*; for further discussion of outcomes more generally, see Glendinning et al, 2006).

Box 4.2: The POETQ approach

The Partnership Outcomes Evaluation Toolkit (POETQ) is a web-based resource that recognises the importance of both process (how well do partners work together?) and outcome (does the partnership make any difference to those who use services?). As a result, POETQ takes a two-pronged approach:

- inviting all staff members to complete an online survey that analyses what is helping/hindering joint work and starts to bring to the surface underpinning assumptions about what outcomes the partnership is aiming to achieve;
- using the information from the staff survey, a research schedule is designed that checks out with service users and carers whether these are the 'right' outcomes to be aiming for and the degree to which the partnership has been successful in changing these outcomes.

In this way, POETQ is both:

- *formative:* it seeks to evaluate how well partners are working together, helps people to understand and make sense of their current context, and highlights both areas for celebration within the partnership as well as areas where development work is needed;
- *summative:* it is evaluative in that it requires partnerships to be explicit about desired outcomes and then analyses the degree to which the partnership is successful in achieving these aims.

For a practical example of POETQ in action, see Dickinson et al's (2013) national evaluation of joint commissioning.

In compiling a list of desired outcomes, it is also important to consider the *type* of outcomes that the partnership is trying to achieve. Typically, many partnerships have (both stated and unstated) outcomes that focus on benefits to service users (better services), benefits for staff (a richer, more satisfying environment) and benefits for the organisation (better use of scarce resources). Perhaps it is this promise of a potential 'win–win' situation that makes partnership such a tempting concept. However, in considering which type of outcome is being sought, it is important to be open and honest. The danger with some partnerships is that they are seeking economic benefits for partners, but dress this up in the language of service user benefits, and this quickly leads to cynicism and disengagement (particularly for service users who typically see straight through such claims; for a practical example, see Dickinson and Glasby, 2010). To aid this process, Mackintosh (1992) provides a helpful distinction between three different types of outcome that a partnership may be trying to achieve:

- *synergy*, bringing together partners with different assets and powers to create something where the whole is greater than the sum of its parts);
- *transformation*, bringing partners together to change the objectives and culture of one or both of the organisations, with the direction of change depending on the power of each individual partner;
- *budget enlargement*, coming together to try to obtain a financial contribution from a third party.

These concepts have since been further developed by Hastings (1996), who provides the typologies set out in Tables 4.1 and 4.2. According to this analysis, Mackintosh's concept of 'synergy' can have a double meaning, referring either to the added value from bringing together and coordinating the resources spent by two or more partners ('resource synergy') or to the new perspectives and innovative solutions that can be created when partners with different cultures and perspectives come together ('policy synergy'). Using these categories, perhaps one of the reasons why partnerships sometimes seem to fail to deliver ambitious aspirations is that service users are seeking the benefits of 'policy synergy' while managers are seeking 'resource synergy'. Or perhaps, as Dickinson et al (2007) illustrate in the case of a Care Trust, while searching for the benefits of 'policy synergy', partnerships may become too concerned with maintaining the rhetoric of peaceful partnership relationships and so inadvertently stifle potentially more innovative approaches in the name of continuity.

In addition, Hastings (1996) also develops Mackintosh's concept of 'transformation', arguing that different things can happen depending on the power balance. Where power is unequal, this can lead to 'uni-directional transformation' (whereby a more powerful partner tries to change the other to become more like itself and where the reluctant, weaker partner is changed against its will). Where both partners accept the need for change and to learn from each other, however, there is the prospect of 'mutual transformation' (whereby all partners change and differences between them begin to reduce).

Table 4.1: Hastings' (1996) definitions of resource and policy synergy

	Process	**Outcome/benefit**
Resource synergy	Cooperation and coordination over the spending of resources	Added value from the resources spent: increased effectiveness or efficiency
Policy synergy	Joint approach developed through combining the different perspectives of each partner	New perspectives/ innovative solutions created

Table 4.2: Hastings' (1996) definitions of transformation

	Process	Result
Uni-directional transformation	One or more partners struggle to modify or to change another partner in their own image. Partners do not accept the need to change themselves	One or more partners change their organisational culture or objectives to become more similar to those of another partner. The transforming partner retains its original style or objectives
Mutual transformation	Reciprocal challenges made to the pre-existing culture and objectives of partners, who seek to learn as well as aspire to teach	All partners involved in the process change to some extent. New sets of objectives, operational styles are developed. Differences between partners are reduced

Understanding what is possible in the current context

While Chapter 2 summarised some of the key frameworks for exploring the extent of 'partnership readiness', other theoretical approaches are also useful when trying to (jointly) understand what is desirable and feasible in the current context. In particular, the literature suggests that it is important to be honest and open about the extent to which different partners are genuinely committed to the outcomes in question (as well as about any pressures that may prevent them from prioritising these issues as much as they would like). Without this, there is a danger that partners sign up enthusiastically to desired outcomes that they will never be able to prioritise in practice, and that the outcomes at stake are not really important enough to all partners to ensure that the necessary action actually materialises. When this happens, it is easy for trust to erode and for faith in the concept of partnership to reduce. To guard against these dangers, the commercial literature emphasises the importance of focusing partnerships on areas that are of importance to both partners (in the case of the private sector, this often means a supplier and a buyer), with successful outcomes much less likely if the partnership is trying to achieve something that is important to only one partner and not the other. Where an issue is not strategically important to both parties, then a contractual relationship (or simply doing it yourself) may be a good way forward (see Figure 4.2 for a helpful summary of this approach).

Figure 4.2: Buyer–supplier strategic perceptions grid

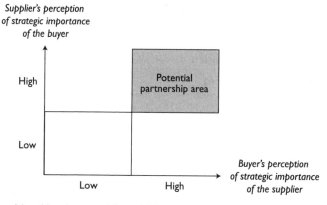

Source: Adapted from Larsson and Bowen (1989, p 221)

At the same time, attempts to explore the current context can benefit from an understanding of the different theoretical approaches to interagency working. While this can be complex, a helpful overview is provided by Sullivan and Skelcher (2002), who distinguish three main schools of thought. As Table 4.3 suggests, optimist approaches assume that partnerships occur through a desire to achieve a shared vision, that collaboration will result in positive outcomes for the whole system and that partners share a level of altruism. In contrast, pessimist approaches see partnership/integration as a means for one organisation to enhance their power at the expense of another. In particular, this pursuit of individual or organisational gain can be focused on achieving a solution that helps the one agency deliver its goals, maintains its power and status, maintains or increases its resources and promotes the agency's view of the world and way of doing things. Finally, a realist perspective concentrates more on the wider environment, and sees partnership/integration as a more pragmatic response to a changing political, economic and social context. As a result, the extent to which partnership will be possible in any given situation may well depend on the mix of motives at work in individual partner agencies and on the extent to which it is possible to harness these different approaches in pursuit of shared and mutually beneficial outcomes.

Table 4.3: Optimist, pessimist and realist approaches to partnership working

	Optimist	Pessimist	Realist
Why collaboration happens?	Achieving shared vision	Maintaining/ enhancing position	Responding to new environments
Key assumptions about other partners	Altruistic	Seeking personal or organisational gain	Realise need to change as society changes
Key factors at work	Role of charismatic leaders/ boundary spanners	Power of individual partners and desire for survival	Ability to adapt to changing environment

Source: Adapted from Sullivan and Skelcher (2002)

Also useful as a means of understanding the current context is a framework for whole systems working initially proposed by Benson (1975) and explored within the context of children's services by Hudson (2004). For Benson, whole systems working depends on the ability to achieve a degree of balance across eight key areas (see Box 4.3). Applying these in practice, Hudson demonstrates how this approach can be a useful tool for conducting a 'health check' on the

—

local whole system, helping to reflect jointly on what is feasible within the current context.

> ### Box 4.3: Benson's (1975) framework for understanding whole systems working
>
> For Benson, it is important to strike a balance between eight different components of the whole system:
>
> - *Domain consensus:* the extent to which there is agreement about the role and scope of each agency's contribution.
> - *Ideological consensus:* the extent to which there is agreement regarding the nature of the tasks facing the partnership.
> - *Positive evaluation:* the extent to which partners have a positive view of each other.
> - *Work coordination:* the extent to which individual partners are prepared to align working patterns.
> - *Fulfilment of programme requirements:* the degree of compatibility between the goals of the partnership and the goals of individual agencies.
> - *Maintenance of a clear domain of high social importance:* the extent to which there is support for the objectives of the partnership from those affected.
> - *Maintenance of resource flows:* the extent to which there is adequate funding for the objectives of the partnership.
> - *Defence of the organisational paradigm:* the extent to which partners see themselves as working for the partnership rather than representing their constituency.
>
> *Source:* Summarised in Hudson (2004, p 9)

How do we get from where we are now to where we want to be?

Once potential partners understand and are clear with each other about what they want to achieve together and about where they are now, the bit in between – what do we do? – ought to be a lot less controversial than is often the case. However, even where partners have used the approach in Figure 4.1 to explore the context and desired outcomes together, it is nearly always issues of structure and process (the 'what do we do?') that generates the most tension. When this happens, some of the frameworks below may help explore the type of relationship and subsequent partnership arrangements that are needed.

In a classic article on 'the five laws of integration', Leutz (1999) argues that health and social care services may need to work together in different ways depending on what they are trying to achieve. This includes three different levels of integration:

- *Linkage:* appropriate for people with mild, moderate or new needs, linkage involves everyone being clear what services exist and how to access them, so that support is provided by autonomous organisations, but systematically linked.
- *Coordination:* with more explicit structures in place, coordination involves being aware of points of tension, confusion and discontinuity in the system and devising policies and procedures for addressing these.
- *Full integration:* for people with complex or unpredictable needs, full integration involves the creation of new services and approaches with a single approach and pooled funding.

In a similar approach, Peck (2002) and Glasby (2005, 2007) challenge partners to consider the balance they need to strike between depth and breadth of relationship in order to achieve desired outcomes (see Figure 4.3). In any given health and social care community, there will be a range of interagency relationships in different places in this matrix, and potential partners may well find it useful to consider what type of relationship they think they need in order to deliver their joint aspirations. Put another way, this framework encourages local organisations to ask themselves a key question about any given piece of interagency working: 'partnership working with whom and for what?'

Figure 4.3: Depth versus breadth of relationship

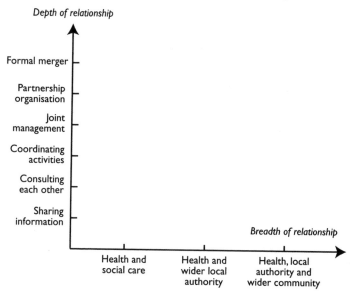

Having explored the depth and breadth of relationship needed to achieve desired outcomes, partners should also consider the different structures and processes they could adopt to make their new partnership arrangements as successful as possible. A helpful contribution is made here by research conducted as part of the national evaluation of former Local Strategic Partnerships (previous forums to provide a cross-cutting focus on the needs of the local area; ODPM, 2005b; see also Glasby and Peck, 2006), which sets out some of the different options with regard to modes of governance, approaches to leadership and levels of engagement from partner agencies (see Boxes 4.4–4.6). While these frameworks offer little by way of answer to some of the complexities surrounding partnership working, they do provide a useful way of categorising different approaches so that potential partners can explore together what kind of relationship they want and how best to organise their subsequent partnership structures. They may also prove useful for new Health and Well-being Boards seeking to learn the lessons of previous strategic partnership bodies. Key questions might therefore include:

- What is the role of the partnership board, and are all partners clear about its primary function (Box 4.4)?
- What is the role of the chair or lead agency, and how can they best balance the different approaches needed in different situations (Box 4.5)?
- What levels of engagement are there around the table, and what balance needs to be struck in order for the partnership to deliver its desired outcomes (Box 4.6)?

Box 4.4: Different modes of governance

- *Advisory:* the board acts as a consultation and discussion forum and often forms the basis for consensus building. It draws its accountability and legitimacy from member organisations, but has no independent power to act.
- *Commissioning:* the partnership has its own staff and authority, is able to implement decisions and commission projects, and therefore has to create its own forms of accountability and legitimacy.
- *Laboratory:* the prime focus is on generating new ideas and new ways of designing local services, drawing on the combined thinking of key stakeholders.
- *Community empowerment:* attention is focused on creating strong networks within the community rather than on the key public agencies.

Source: ODPM (2005b)

Box 4.5: Different approaches to leadership

- *Holding the chair:* setting agendas, managing the business, working the board towards decisions, ensuring that all stakeholders can express their views.
- *Committing partners:* generating collective ownership of and commitment to the partnership from key leaders in partner organisations, establishing accountability to the partnership through influence.
- *Role modelling:* behaving as if joint working matters, respecting diversity, modelling collaboration.
- *Representation:* taking partnership business back into one's own organisation and ensuring that others provide back-up and that the organisation fulfils the partnership's expectations of it.

Source: ODPM (2005b)

Box 4.6: Different levels of engagement

- *Defensive participation:* often new to partnership working, such organisations are concerned about the perceived resource implications or threat of participation – their presence is often defensive (to ensure that their agency does not 'lose out').
- *Opportunistic participation:* such organisations may not see the partnership as core to their own objectives, but are able to see and grasp potential benefits opportunistically. This type of partner is often seen as taking more from the partnership than it contributes.
- *Active participation:* such organisations are strongly committed to the partnership and see taking part as a natural extension of their repertoire for tackling items on their own agenda, as well as those of other partners.

Source: ODPM (2005b)

Overall, this chapter has sought to provide an overview of some key frameworks that may help to explore the scope for more integrated care and to design partnerships that deliver desired outcomes. Central to this process is the ability to hold back from debates about structure and about process. Partnerships and integrated services are only ever a means to an end, and service users, practitioners, managers, policy makers and researchers all have a duty to make sure that they never become an end in themselves.

Reflective exercises

1. Think about a partnership or integrated approach where you live or work. Using the context-process-outcome framework in Figure 4.1 above, is it clear (to all partners involved) what services are trying to achieve, and have they designed their subsequent partnership/joint approach in such a way that helps them move from where they were to where they want to be? What could they have done differently, and was a 'partnership' the best way forward?

2. Reflecting on recent government policy, what are policy makers trying to achieve from promoting more integrated approaches? Do the Hastings frameworks in Tables 4.1 and 4.2 help to develop your thinking and help to critique the initial policy?

3. Choose a local integrated service or partnership. Using the framework in Figure 4.2, do both partners have equal levels of commitment, and was a partnership the best way forward?

4. Reflecting on the possible motives of the different partners involved, to what extent is it possible to see elements of the optimist, pessimist and realist approaches set out in Table 4.3?

5. Using Leutz's categories of linkage, coordination and full integration and/or Peck's model of depth versus breadth, map local partnerships. To what extent do local partners have the right level of relationship with the right organisations in order to achieve desired outcomes?

---

6. For those involved in Health and Well-being Boards or other strategic partnership forums, what insights do the concepts in Boxes 4.4-4.6 provide? Do you have the 'right' board, leadership and engagement for what you are trying to achieve?

Further reading and resources

Many of the key texts for this chapter are summarised in the relevant sections above. However:

- For a summary of key theoretical approaches to partnership working, see Sullivan and Skelcher's (2002) *Working across boundaries*. Dickinson and Glasby's (2010) 'Why partnership doesn't work' develops some of this initial material further and builds on the concepts summarised above in Table 4.3.
- For more detail on evaluating outcomes in interagency settings, see Helen Dickinson's (2008) book in the present series, *Evaluating outcomes in health and social care*.

5

Recommendations for policy and practice

Ultimately, the questions, summaries and frameworks set out in this book lead us to highlight a series of practical recommendations and potential warnings, both for policy and for practice.

For policy makers:

- Resist the temptation to look for structural 'solutions' – these often just give a false impression of change and can make things worse rather than better.
- A key role for government is to be clear about desired outcomes and to hold local areas to account for achieving these. How best to deliver such outcomes will vary from area to area, and local leaders need the flexibility to do what will work best for their area.
- Policy makers often use the language of partnership or integration, but greater clarity is needed as to what these phrases actually mean. A key question to ask is if partnership is the answer, what was the question?
- When seeking to compel the creation of a partnership, it is important to blend elements of hierarchy, market and network in order to maximise the chances of success.
- Greater research is required to understand the extent to which partnerships really do lead to better outcomes (and, if so, what kinds of partnership, for whom and under what circumstances).
- While the current emphasis on evidence-based practice is welcome, this needs to be broadened so that we also learn from 'what does not work', so that we learn from current policy/practice and so that we

view service user experiences and practitioner wisdom as potentially valid sources of evidence.
- The current policy and financial climate could make the delivery of integrated care even harder, and this could lead to a growing mismatch between policy rhetoric and reality at ground level.

For local organisations and frontline services:

- There is a need to be clearer in our use of language so that terms such as 'partnership working' and 'integrated care' are used more precisely, and so that all local partners have the same understanding of what is being proposed.
- Local partners need to focus first on desired outcomes, before moving on to consider the current context. Issues of process and structure (the 'what do we do?') should come last, and only when we have a jointly agreed understanding of where we are now and where we are trying to get to.
- While some form of partnership may be the best way forward, this is not automatically the case, and a more critical approach to partnership working may well be needed.
- When asked to work in partnership, always consider who you need to work with and how in order to achieve desired outcomes.
- When designing local partnership arrangements, it is important to reflect carefully on the type of partnership you need, the prime roles it will need to fulfil, the type of leadership it needs and the motives/levels of engagement of key partners.
- While it can sometimes be helpful to be ambitious in scope, it can also be necessary to consider what is feasible in the current context.
- In the current context, Health and Well-being Boards could helpfully learn from previous strategic partnership forums (such as Local Strategic Partnerships). Although clinical commissioning offers new opportunities for joint work, the relationship between social care and general practice is starting from a low base.

Above all, we believe that partnership and integration are here to stay (even if the exact language used changes over time). For all the complexities explored in this book, it seems increasingly clear that single agencies cannot respond sufficiently to the complexity of need that is out there – especially in challenging financial circumstances. Policy may not be clear what it means by concepts such as 'partnership' or 'integrated care', and such approaches are frequently portrayed as a 'good thing' (without anyone being clear exactly how and why). Calling something a partnership is also much easier than actually trying to join up a system that was designed on a silo basis, and creating something that feels integrated to people on the receiving end (which is surely an acid test). However, doing some things together makes sense intuitively, and we know all too well what can happen if services aren't sufficiently joined-up. In future, perhaps the trick is to be a little more healthily sceptical about when partnership/integration is the right solution, but also to keep on believing. Perhaps it is because partnerships and integration are so important that we need to use them sparingly, always seeing them as a means to an end and never as an end in themselves.

References

6, P., Leat, D., Seltzer, K. and Stoker, G. (2002) *Towards holistic governance*, Basingstoke: Palgrave.

6, P., Goodwin, N., Peck, E. and Freeman, T. (2006) *Managing networks of twenty-first century organisations*, Basingstoke: Palgrave.

Audit Commission (1998) *A fruitful partnership: Effective partnership working*, London: Audit Commission.

Audit Commission (2002) *Integrated services for older people*, London: Audit Commission.

Audit Commission (2005) *Governing partnerships: Bridging the accountability gap*, London: Audit Commission.

Baggott, R. (2007) *Understanding health policy*, Bristol: The Policy Press.

Balloch, S. and Taylor, M. (eds) (2001) *Partnership working: Policy and practice*, Bristol: The Policy Press.

Banks, P. (2002) *Partnerships under pressure: A commentary on progress in partnership working between the NHS and local government*, London: The King's Fund.

Barnes, M., Bauld, L., Benzeval, M., Judge, K., Mackenzie, M. and Sullivan, H. (2005) *Health Action Zones: Partnerships for equity*, London: Routledge.

Barrett, G., Sellman, D. and Thomas, J. (eds) (2005) *Interprofessional working in health and social care*, Basingstoke: Palgrave.

Barton, P., Bryan, S. and Glasby, J., Hewitt, G., Jagger, C., Kaambwa, B., Graham, M., Nancarrow, S., Parker, H. and Parker, S. (2006) *A national evaluation of the costs and outcomes of intermediate care for older people*, Birmingham/Leicester: Health Services Management Centre and Leicester Nuffield Research Unit.

Batty, D. (2003) 'The end of the affair: row over strategy splits joint management partnership', *The Guardian*, 3 September (www.politics.guardian.co.uk, accessed 20/04/2007).

BBC (2003) 'Trusts to take over child care', 28 January (www.bbc.co.uk, accessed 19/02/2007).

BBC (2005) '"Home alone" deaths for thousands', 29 December (www. bbc.co.uk, accessed 16/02/2007).

Belsky, J., Barnes, J. and Melhuish, E. (eds) (2007) *The national evaluation of Sure Start: Does area-based early intervention work?*, Bristol: The Policy Press.

Benson, J.K. (1975) 'The inter-organisational network as a political economy', *Administrative Science Quarterly*, vol 20, pp 229-49.

Britnell, M. (2007) 'A freedom framework will unite former foes', *Health Service Journal*, 1 February, pp 18-19.

Buse, K., Mays, N. and Walt, G. (2005) *Making health policy*, Maidenhead: Open University Press.

Cameron, A. and Lart, R. (2003) 'Factors promoting and obstacles hindering joint working: a systematic review of the research evidence', *Journal of Integrated Care*, vol 11, issue 2, pp 9-17.

Cameron, A., Lart, R., Bostock, L. and Coomber, C. (2012) *Factors that promote and hinder joint and integrated working between health and social care services*, Research Briefing 41, London: Social Care Institute for Excellence.

Carpenter, J. and Dickinson, H. (2008) *Interprofessional education and training*, Bristol: The Policy Press.

CHI (Commission for Health Improvement) (2003) *Investigation into matters arising from care on Rowan Ward, Manchester Mental Health and Social Care Trust*, London: CHI (now the Care Quality Commission).

Connell, J.P. and Kubisch, A.C. (1998) 'Applying a theory of change approach to the evaluation of comprehensive community initiatives: progress, prospects and problems', in K. Fulbright-Anderson, A.C. Kubisch, and J.P. Connell (eds) *New approaches to evaluating community initiatives: Volume 2 – Theory, measurement and analysis*, Washington, DC: The Aspen Institute.

Coopers & Lybrand (1993) *Making a success of acquisitions*, London: Coopers & Lybrand.

CQC (Care Quality Commission) (2012) 'National report finds half of learning disability services did not meet standards', CQC press release, 25 June (www.cqc.org.uk/media/national-report-finds-half-learning-disability-services-did-not-meet-standards).

Craig, G. and Manthorpe, J. (1999) *Unfinished business? Local government reorganisation and social services*, Bristol: The Policy Press in association with the Joseph Rowntree Foundation.

CSCI (Commission for Social Care Inspection) (2004) *Leaving hospital – The price of delays*, London: CSCI.

CSCI (2005) *Leaving hospital – Revisited*, London: CSCI.

Curry, N. and Ham, C. (2010) *Clinical and service integration: The route to improved outcomes*, London: The King's Fund.

DH (Department of Health) (1998) *Partnership in action: New opportunities for joint working between health and social services – A discussion document*, London: DH.

DH (2000) *The NHS plan: A plan for investment, a plan for reform*, London: The Stationery Office.

DH (2001) *Valuing people: A new strategy for learning disability for the 21st century*, London: The Stationery Office.

DH (2006) *Our health, our care, our say*, London: The Stationery Office.

DH (2010) *Equity and excellence: Liberating the NHS*, London: The Stationery Office.

DH (2013) *Integrated care: Our shared commitment*, London: DH.

Dickinson, H. (2006) 'The evaluation of health and social care partnerships: an analysis of approaches and synthesis for the future', *Health and Social Care in the Community*, vol 14, no 5, pp 375-83.

Dickinson, H. (2008) *Evaluating outcomes in health and social care*, Bristol: The Policy Press.

Dickinson, H. and Glasby, J. (2010) 'Why partnership working doesn't work: pitfalls, problems and possibilities in English health and social care', *Public Management Review*, vol 12, no 6, pp 811-28.

Dickinson, H., Peck, E. and Davidson, D. (2007) 'Opportunity seized or missed? A case study of leadership and organisational change in the creation of a care trust', *Journal of Interprofessional Care*, vol 21, no 5, pp 503-13.

Dickinson, H., Peck, E. and Smith, J. (2006) *Leadership in organisational transition – What can we learn from research evidence? Summary report*, Birmingham: Health Services Management Centre.

Dickinson, H., Glasby, J., Nicholds, A., Jeffares, S., Robinson, S. and Sullivan, H. (2013) *Joint commissioning in health and social care: An exploration of definitions, processes, services and outcomes*, Birmingham: Health Services Management Centre (for the NHS Health Service Research and Delivery programme).

Dowling, B., Powell, M. and Glendinning, C. (2004) 'Conceptualising successful partnerships', *Health and Social Care in the Community*, vol 12, no 4, pp 309-17.

Edwards, A., Barnes, M., Plewis, I. and Morris, K. et al (2006) *Working to prevent the social exclusion of children and young people: Final lessons from the national evaluation of the Children's Fund*, Birmingham: Department for Education and Skills, University of Birmingham.

Edwards, N. (2010) *The triumph of hope over experience: Lessons from the history of reorganisation*, London: NHS Confederation.

Ellins, J. and Glasby, J. (2008) *Implementing joint strategic needs assessment: Pitfalls, possibilities and progress*, Leeds: Integrated Care Network/Health Services Management Centre.

Farnsworth, A. (2012) 'Unintended consequences? The impact of NHS reforms upon Torbay Care Trust', *Journal of Integrated Care*, vol 20, no 3, pp 146-51.

Field, J. and Peck, E. (2003) 'Mergers and acquisitions in the private sector: what are the lessons for health and social services?', *Social Policy and Administration*, vol 37, no 7, pp 742-55.

Fraser, D. (2003) *The evolution of the British welfare state* (3rd edn), Basingstoke: Palgrave.

Fulop, N., Protopsaltis, G., King, A., Allen, P., Hutchings, A. and Normand, C. (2005) 'Changing organisations: a study of the context and processes of mergers of health care providers in England', *Social Science and Medicine*, vol 60, no 1, pp 119-30.

Fulop, N., Protopsaltis, G., Hutchings, A., King, A., Allen, P., Normand, C. and Walters, R. (2002) 'Process and impact of mergers of NHS trust: multicentre case study and management cost analysis', *British Medical Journal*, vol 325, pp 246-52.

Glasby, J. (2003) *Hospital discharge: Integrating health and social care*, Abingdon: Radcliffe Medical Press.

—

Glasby, J. (2004) *Working together to meet the needs of people with learning disabilities: A report of a national workshop*, Birmingham: Health Services Management Centre/Valuing People Support Team.

Glasby, J. (2005) 'The integration dilemma: how deep and how broad to go?', *Journal of Integrated Care*, vol 13, no 5, pp 27-30.

Glasby, J. (2012a) *Understanding health and social care* (2nd edn), Bristol: The Policy Press.

Glasby, J. (ed) (2012b) *Evidence, policy and practice: Critical perspectives in health and social care*, Bristol: The Policy Press.

Glasby, J. and Beresford, P. (2006) 'Who knows best? Evidence-based practice and the service user contribution', *Critical Social Policy*, vol 26, no 1, pp 268-84.

Glasby, J. and Dickinson, H. (eds) (2009) *International perspectives on health and social care: Partnership working in action*, Oxford: Blackwell-Wiley

Glasby, J. and Littlechild, R. (2004) *The health and social care divide: The experiences of older people* (2nd edn), Bristol: The Policy Press.

Glasby, J. and Littlechild, R. (2009) *Direct payments and personal budgets: Putting personalisation into practice* (2nd edn), Bristol: The Policy Press.

Glasby, J. and Peck, E. (eds) (2003) *Care trusts: Partnership working in action*, Abingdon: Radcliffe Medical Press.

Glasby, J. and Peck, E. (2006) *We have to stop meeting like this: The governance of inter-agency partnerships*, Leeds: Integrated Care Network.

Glasby, J., Dickinson, H. and Miller, R. (2011) *All in this together? Making best use of health and social care resources in an era of austerity*, Policy Paper No 9, Birmingham: Health Services Management Centre.

Glasby, J., Miller, R. and Posaner, R. (forthcoming) *New conversations with new players? The relationship between primary care and social care in an era of clinical commissioning*, Birmingham: Health Services Management Centre/School for Social Care Research.

Glasby, J., Walshe, K. and Harvey, G. (eds) (2007) 'What counts as "evidence" in "evidence-based practice"?', special edition of *Evidence & Policy*, vol 3, no 3.

Glendinning, C., Powell, M. and Rummery, K. (eds) (2002a) *Partnerships, New Labour and the governance of welfare*, Bristol: The Policy Press.

—

Glendinning, C., Hudson, B., Hardy, B. and Young, R. (2002b) *National evaluation of notifications for the use of the Section 31 partnership flexibilities in the Health Act 1999: Final project report*, Leeds/Manchester: Nuffield Institute for Health/National Primary Care Research and Development Centre.

Glendinning, C., Coleman, A. and Rummery, K. (2002c) 'Partnerships, performance and primary care: developing integrated services for older people in England', *Ageing & Society*, vol 22, pp 185-208.

Glendinning, C., Clarke, S., Hare, P., Kotchetkova, I., Maddison, J. and Newbronner, L. (2006) *Outcomes-focused services for older people*, London: Social Care Institute for Excellence.

Godfrey, M., Keen, J., Townsend, J., Moore, J., Ware, P., Hardy, B., West, R., Weatherly, H. and Henderson, C. (2005) *An evaluation of intermediate care for older people: Final report*, Leeds: University of Leeds.

Godfrey, M., Townsend, J., Cornes, M., Donaghy, E., Hubbard, G. and Manthorpe, J. (2008) *Reimbursement in practice: The last piece of the jigsaw? A comparative study of delayed hospital discharge in England and Scotland*, Stirling, Leeds and London: University of Stirling, University of Leeds, King's College London.

Goodwin, N., Smith, J., Davies, A., Perry, C., Rosen, R., Dixon, A., Dixon, J. and Ham, C. (2012) *Integrated care for patients and populations: Improving outcomes by working together*, London: The King's Fund.

Greig, R. (2000) 'The locality learning disability service', Paper presented to the Community Care Development Centre/King's College London Conference on 'Community Learning Disability Teams', 13 December, London.

Greig, R. and Poxton, R. (2001) 'From joint commissioning to partnership working – will the new policy framework make a difference?', *Managing Community Care*, vol 9, no 4, pp 32-8.

Hardy, B., Hudson, B. and Waddington, E. (2003) *Assessing strategic partnership: The Partnership Assessment Tool*, London: Office of the Deputy Prime Minister/Nuffield Institute for Health.

Hastings, A. (1996) 'Unravelling the process of "partnership" in urban regeneration policy', *Urban Studies*, vol 33, no 2, pp 253-68.

—

Healthcare Commission/CSCI (Commission for Social Care Inspection) (2006) *Joint investigation into the provision of services for people with learning disabilities at Cornwall Partnership NHS Trust*, London: Healthcare Commission.

Health Service Journal (2006) 'Government launches media offensive amid £500m deficit', *Health Service Journal*, 8 June, p 5.

Henwood, M. (2004) *Reimbursement and delayed discharges*, Leeds: Integrated Care Network.

Henwood, M. (2006) 'Effective partnership working: a case study of hospital discharge', *Health and Social Care in the Community*, vol 14, no 5, pp 400-7.

Hill, M. (2000) *Understanding social policy* (6th edn), Oxford: Blackwell.

Hill, M. (2004) *The public policy process* (4th edn), Harlow: Pearson Education.

HM Treasury (2003) *Every child matters*, London: The Stationery Office.

Hudson, B. (2000) 'Inter-agency collaboration: a sceptical view', in A. Brechin, H. Brown and M.A. Eby (eds) *Critical practice in health and social care*, Milton Keynes: Open University Press.

Hudson, B. (2002) 'Integrated care and structural change in England: the case of care trusts', *Policy Studies*, vol 23, no 2, pp 77-95.

Hudson, B. (2004) *Whole systems working*, Leeds: Integrated Care Network.

Humphries, R., Galea, A., Sonola, L. and Mundle, C. (2012) *Health and Wellbeing Boards: System leaders or talking shops?*, London: The King's Fund.

Huntingdon, J. (1981) *Social work and general medical practice: Collaboration or conflict?*, London: Allen & Unwin.

Jelphs, K. and Dickinson, H. (2008) *Working in teams*, Bristol: The Policy Press.

Johri, M., Béland, F. and Bergman, H. (2003) 'International experiments in integrated care for the elderly: a synthesis of the evidence', *International Journal of Geriatric Psychiatry*, vol 18, pp 222-35.

Jupp, B. (2000) *Working together: Creating a better environment for cross-sector partnerships*, London: Demos.

Kodner, D. (2006) 'Whole system approaches to health and social care partnerships for the frail elderly: an exploration of North American models and lessons', *Health and Social Care in the Community*, vol 14, no 5, pp 384-90.

Laming, H. (2003) *The Victoria Climbié inquiry*, London: The Stationery Office.

Laming, H. (2009) *The protection of children in England: A progress report*, London: The Stationery Office.

Larsson, R. and Bowen, D.E. (1989) 'Organization and customer: managing design and coordination of services', *Academy of Management Review*, vol 14, no 2, pp 213-33.

Leathard, A. (ed) (1994) *Going inter-professional: Working together for health and welfare*, Hove: Routledge.

Leichsenring, K. and Alaszewski, A. (eds) (2004) *Providing integrated health and social care for older persons: A European overview of issues at stake*, Aldershot: Ashgate.

Leutz, W. (1999) 'Five laws for integrating medical and social services: lessons from the United States and the United Kingdom', *The Milbank Quarterly*, vol 77, no 1, pp 77-110.

Ling, T. (2000) 'Unpacking partnership: the case of health', in J. Clarke and S.M.E. Gewirtz (eds) *New managerialism, new welfare?*, London: Sage Publications.

McCoy, D., Godden, S., Pollock, A.M. and Bianchessi, C. (2007) 'Carrot and sticks? The Community Care Act (2003) and the effect of financial incentives on delays in discharge from hospitals in England', *Journal of Public Health*, vol 29, no 3, pp 281-27.

McCulloch, A. and Parker, C. (2004) 'Inquiries, assertive outreach and compliance: is there a relationship?', in N. Stanley and J. Manthorpe (eds) *The age of the inquiry: Learning and blaming in health and social care*, London: Routledge.

Mackintosh, M. (1992) 'Partnership: issues of policy and negotiation', *Local Economy*, vol 7, no 3, pp 210-24.

Manthorpe, J., Cornes, M., Rapaport, J., Moriaty, J., Bright, L., Clough, R. and Iliffe, S. (2006) 'Commissioning community well-being: focus on older people and transport', *Journal of Integrated Care*, vol 14, no 4, pp 28-37.

Markwell, S., Watson, J., Speller, V., Platt, S. and Younger, T. (2003) *The working partnership*, London: Health Development Agency (now NICE).

Meads, G. and Ashcroft, J., with Barr, H., Scott, R. and Wild, A. (2005) *The case for interprofessional collaboration in health and social care*, Oxford: Blackwell.

Means, R. and Smith, R. (1998) *From Poor Law to community care*, Basingstoke: Macmillan.

Means, R., Richards, S. and Smith, R. (2003) *Community care: Policy and practice* (3rd edn), Basingstoke: Palgrave.

Miller, R., Dickinson, H. and Glasby, J. (2011) *The vanguard of integration or a lost tribe? Care trusts ten years on*, Birmingham: Health Services Management Centre.

NHS Future Forum (2012) *Integration: A report from the NHS Future Forum*, London: NHS Future Forum.

ODPM (Office of the Deputy Prime Minister) (2005a) *A process evaluation of the negotiation of pilot local area agreements*, London: ODPM.

ODPM (2005b) *Evaluation of local strategic partnerships: Interim report*, London: ODPM.

ODPM (2007) *Evidence of savings, improved outcomes, and good practice attributed to local area agreements*, London: ODPM.

ODPM and Department of Transport (2006) *National evaluation of local strategic partnerships: Formative evaluation and action research programme, 2002-2005*, London: ODPM.

O'Hara, M. (2006) 'Pain but no gain', *The Guardian*, 10 May (www.politics.guardian.co.uk, accessed 20/04/2007).

O'Keeffe, M., Hills, A., Doyle, M., McCreadie, C., Scholes, S., Constantine, R., Tinker, A., Manthorpe, J., Biggs, S. and Erens, B. (2007) *UK study of abused and neglect of older people: Prevalence survey report*, London: National Centre for Social Research.

Pawson, R. and Tilley, N. (1997) *Realistic evaluation*, London: Sage Publications.

Payne, M. (2000) *Teamwork in mutliprofessional care*, Basingstoke: Macmillan.

Peck, E. (2002) 'Integrating health and social care', *Managing Community Care*, vol 10, no 3, pp 16-19.

Peck, E. and Dickinson, H. (2008) *Managing and leading in inter-agency settings*, Bristol: The Policy Press.

Peck, E. and Freeman, T. (2005) *Reconfiguring PCTs: Influences and options* (briefing paper prepared for the NHS Alliance), Birmingham: Health Services Management Centre.

Peck, E. and 6, P. (2006) *Beyond delivery: Policy implementation as sense-making and settlement*, Basingstoke: Palgrave Macmillan.

Peck, E., Gulliver, P. and Towell, D. (2002) *Modernising partnerships: Evaluation of Somerset's innovations in the commissioning and organisation of mental health services – Final report*, London: Institute for Applied Health and Social Policy, King's College London.

Perkins, N., Smith, K., Hunter, D.J., Bambra, C. and Joyce, K. (2010) '"What counts is what works"? New Labour and partnerships in public health', *Policy & Politics*, vol 38, no 1, pp 101-17.

Pollard, K., Thomas, J. and Miers, M. (eds) (2010) *Understanding interprofessional working in health and social care*, Basingstoke: Palgrave.

Powell, M. and Dowling, B. (2006) 'New Labour's partnerships: comparing conceptual models with existing forms', *Social Policy and Society*, vol 5, no 2, pp 305-14.

RAND Europe/Ernst & Young (2012) *National evaluation of the Department of Health's integrated care pilots*, Cambridge: RAND Europe.

Rodríguez, C., Langley, A., Béland, F. and Denis, J.-L. (2007) 'Governance, power, and mandated collaboration in an interorganizational network', *Administration and Society*, vol 39, no 2, pp 150-93.

Rummery, K. and Glendinning, C. (2000) *Primary care and social services: Developing new partnerships for older people*, Abingdon: Radcliffe Medical Press.

Rycroft-Malone, J., Seers, K., Titchen, A., Harvey, G., Kitson, A. and McCormack, B. (2004) 'What counts as evidence in evidence-based practice?', *Journal of Advanced Nursing*, vol 47, no 1, pp 81-90.

Skelcher, C., Mathur, N. and Smith, M. (2004) *Effective partnership and good governance: Lessons for policy and practice*, Birmingham: Institute of Local Government Studies, University of Birmingham.

SSI (Social Services Inspectorate)/Audit Commission (2004) *Old virtues, new virtues: An overview of the changes in social care services over the seven years of Joint Reviews in England, 1996-2003*, London: SSI/Audit Commission.

Sullivan, H. and Skelcher, C. (2002) *Working across boundaries: Collaboration in public services*, Basingstoke: Palgrave.

Thistlethwaite, P. (2011) *Integrating health and social care in Torbay: Improving care for Mrs Smith*, London: The King's Fund.

Thomson, A.M. and Perry, J.L. (1998) 'Can AmeriCorps build communities?', *Nonprofit and Voluntary Sector Quarterly*, vol 27, no 4, pp 399-420.

Thompson, G., Frances, J., Levacic, R. and Mitchell, J. (1991) *Markets, hierarchies and networks: The coordination of social life*, London: Sage Publications in association with The Open University.

Timmins, N. (2012) *Never again? The story of the Health and Social Care Act 2012*, London: The King's Fund.

University of East Anglia (2007) *Children's trust pathfinders: Innovative partnerships for improving the well-being of children and young people*, Norwich: University of East Anglia in association with the National Children's Bureau.

Walshe, K. (2003) 'Foundation hospitals: a new direction for NHS reform', *Journal of the Royal Society of Medicine*, vol 96, pp 106-10.

Welsh Assembly Government (2011) *Sustainable social services for Wales: A framework for action*, Cardiff: Welsh Assembly Government.

Wistow, G. and Waddington, E. (2006) 'Learning from doing: implications of the Barking and Dagenham experiences for integrating health and social care', *Journal of Integrated Care*, vol 14, pp 8-18.

Index